ATKINS DIET

FOR

EPILEPSY

100+ Transformative Recipes and Nutritional Strategies for Seizure Management and Improved Well-being

Kingsley Klopp

To show our appreciation for your purchase, we're delighted to offer you these special bonuses as a heartfelt thank you

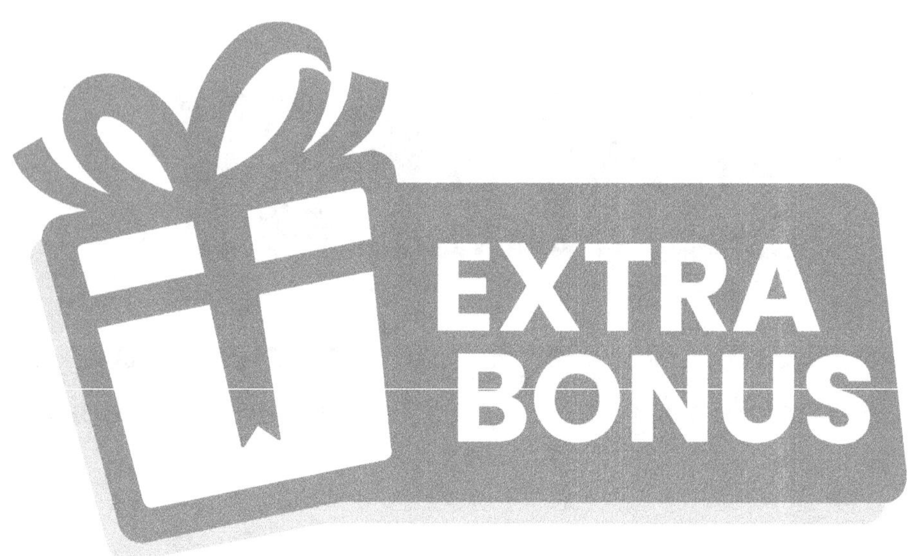

1. A Food Tracker Journal
2. Downloadable E-BOOK featuring full-color images of finished recipes

Table of Content

Poultry Recipes

Important Note

First and foremost, thank you for choosing **Atkins Diet for Epilepsy**. We are thrilled to embark on this journey with you, offering delicious, carefully crafted recipes designed to support your health and well-being.

However, as you turn the pages and begin to explore the myriad of culinary delights within this book, we feel it is important to share a gentle reminder. Each of us is unique, with individual dietary needs and health conditions that require personalized attention. While the recipes in this cookbook are designed to be nutritious and supportive for those managing epilepsy, it is essential to recognize that one size does not fit all. Your body's response to certain foods can be as individual as your fingerprint. What works wonders for one person may not have the same effect for another. Therefore, we encourage you to listen to your body and adjust these recipes to better suit your personal dietary needs and preferences. Don't hesitate to experiment with ingredient substitutions and portion sizes that align with your nutritional goals and tolerances.

Moreover, navigating dietary changes, especially for medical conditions like epilepsy, can sometimes be daunting. If at any point you find yourself feeling uncertain or confused, please seek the guidance of your healthcare provider. Consulting with your doctor or a registered dietitian can provide you with the tailored advice and reassurance you need to move forward confidently and safely.

It's also important to note that the nutritional information provided in this cookbook is approximate. Variations in ingredients, brands, and preparation methods can lead to differences in the final nutritional content of your meals. These figures are intended to serve as a helpful guide rather than an absolute measure. Always consider the specific products you use and, if necessary, consult nutrition labels to ensure you're meeting your dietary needs.

Furthermore, If our cookbook has brought joy to your kitchen and table, we'd be thrilled to hear about your experiences in an Amazon review. On the flip side, if you stumble upon any hiccups while exploring our recipes, don't hesitate to get in touch at **kloppkingsley@gmail.com.**

In creating this cookbook, our aim was to blend professional insights with a personal touch, recognizing that every journey with epilepsy is deeply personal and unique. We hope that the recipes inspire you, bring joy to your meals, and support your health in meaningful ways. Remember, you are not alone on this path. There is a community of people, including healthcare professionals and fellow readers, ready to support you every step of the way.

Introduction.

Imagine a life where the fear of the next seizure doesn't loom over every moment, where your days aren't dictated by the unpredictability of epilepsy. Picture a world where you have more control over your health, where you can make choices that empower you, reduce your seizure frequency, and improve your overall quality of life. This is not a far-fetched dream. This is a possibility that the Atkins Diet for Epilepsy can bring into your reality. Welcome to **Atkins Diet for Epilepsy,** a comprehensive guide that promises to transform the way you think about epilepsy management. Whether you're newly diagnosed or have been navigating the turbulent waters of epilepsy for years, this book is designed to be your compass, leading you toward a path of fewer seizures and greater well-being.

You might be wondering, "Why the Atkins Diet?" The Atkins Diet, renowned for its effectiveness in weight loss and metabolic health, has an incredible yet less publicized potential: it can significantly help manage epilepsy. Research has shown that a low-carbohydrate, high-fat diet can alter brain metabolism in a way that reduces seizure activity. This isn't just about cutting carbs or losing weight; it's about reclaiming your life from the grip of epilepsy. Let's start with a bit of history. The ketogenic diet, a precursor to the Atkins Diet, has been used since the 1920s to treat epilepsy. It's a diet that forces the body to burn fats rather than carbohydrates, producing ketones which have a stabilizing effect on the brain's electrical activity. The Atkins Diet shares this principle but offers a more palatable and sustainable approach for many people. Imagine a diet where you can enjoy rich, savory foods like avocado, cheese, nuts, and even bacon, all while managing your epilepsy. It sounds too good to be true, but it's not. In this book, we will journey through the science behind the Atkins Diet and its effects on epilepsy. We'll explore the different types of seizures and how dietary changes can impact their frequency and severity. You will learn about the foundational principles of the Atkins Diet, how it differs from and aligns with the ketogenic diet, and why it might be the perfect fit for you.

But this book isn't just about theory. It's a practical guide to transforming your diet and, by extension, your life. We'll walk you through meal planning, grocery shopping, and meal prepping, ensuring you're equipped with the tools you need to succeed. We'll also delve into the emotional and psychological aspects of living with epilepsy and how dietary changes can influence your mental health and overall sense of well-being.

One of the most compelling aspects of the Atkins Diet for Epilepsy is its focus on sustainable change. We know that drastic diet changes can be overwhelming and hard to maintain. That's why this book emphasizes gradual shifts, helping you transition smoothly into a low-carb lifestyle without feeling deprived or stressed. You'll find delicious, easy-to-follow recipes that will make you look forward to your meals. Think creamy spinach, hearty lasagna, succulent grilled fish, and decadent desserts that won't spike your blood sugar or your seizure threshold. Community and support are also integral parts of this journey. We encourage you to engage with others who are on the same path. Share your successes, discuss your challenges, and celebrate the milestones together. Remember, you are not alone in this; there's a whole community cheering you on.

By the end of this book, you will not only understand the Atkins Diet and its potential to manage epilepsy but also feel confident in your ability to implement it in your life. You will be armed with knowledge, practical tips, and a newfound hope that managing epilepsy is within your control. This isn't just a diet; it's a lifestyle change that could significantly reduce your seizures and enhance your quality of life.

So, are you ready to take the first step towards a brighter, more stable future? Dive in, explore the pages of this book, and begin your journey toward seizure freedom with the **Atkins Diet for Epilepsy.** Your path to better health starts here.

Part 1

Understanding Epilepsy

What is Epilepsy?

Epilepsy is more than just a medical condition; it's a complex and often misunderstood journey that millions of people worldwide navigate daily. At its core, epilepsy is a neurological disorder characterized by recurrent, unprovoked seizures. But behind this clinical definition lies a tapestry of human experiences, fears, and hopes that shape the lives of those affected. Imagine, for a moment, the sudden onset of a storm. A clear sky darkens without warning, lightning flashes, and thunder roars. This is what a seizure can feel like for someone with epilepsy—a sudden, uncontrollable surge of electrical activity in the brain that disrupts the normal patterns and rhythms of their thoughts, feelings, and actions. Epilepsy is not a one-size-fits-all condition; it manifests uniquely in each person it touches. For some, seizures are brief and infrequent, a distant rumble in an otherwise calm life. For others, they are a relentless tempest, a constant and unpredictable force that shapes every decision and moment. This variability can make epilepsy a particularly isolating experience, as those affected often feel that no one truly understands what they are going through.

The impact of epilepsy extends far beyond the seizures themselves. The uncertainty and unpredictability of when a seizure might occur can cast a shadow over daily life, affecting everything from personal relationships to professional aspirations. The fear of having a seizure in public, of being judged or misunderstood, can lead to social withdrawal and a profound sense of isolation. But amidst the challenges, there is also resilience. Many people with epilepsy and their families show remarkable strength and adaptability. They learn to recognize the subtle signs that a seizure might be coming, develop strategies to minimize triggers, and find ways to live full, meaningful lives despite the hurdles they face. Epilepsy is also a story of hope and progress. Advances in medical research and treatment options are continually improving the quality of life for those with the condition. New medications, dietary therapies like the Atkins Diet, and even surgical interventions offer promising avenues for better seizure control and overall health. The growing awareness and understanding of epilepsy in society are also helping to break down the stigma and misconceptions that have long surrounded it.

In the heart of epilepsy lies a powerful narrative of human spirit. It is a testament to the courage of those who face each day with the possibility of a seizure, yet refuse to let it define them. It is a call to empathy for those of us who may not fully understand but can offer support, kindness, and acceptance. And it is a beacon of hope that, through continued research and compassion, we can create a world where epilepsy is not a barrier to living one's best life. In recognizing and embracing the full humanity of those affected by epilepsy, we can turn a clinical diagnosis into a story of triumph, connection, and unyielding hope.

Types of Epilepsy and Seizures

Types of Epilepsy

1. **Focal (Partial) Epilepsy**
   - Focal Onset Aware Seizures (Simple Partial Seizures): These seizures originate in a specific area of the brain and do not affect consciousness. Symptoms can include involuntary movements, sensory disturbances, or a sense of déjà vu.
   - Focal Onset Impaired Awareness Seizures (Complex Partial Seizures): These seizures also start in a localized region of the brain but affect awareness and consciousness. Individuals may exhibit repetitive movements, stare blankly, or have difficulty responding to their environment.

2. **Generalized Epilepsy**
   - Absence Seizures (Petit Mal Seizures): Characterized by brief, sudden lapses in consciousness, absence seizures are often mistaken for daydreaming. These seizures are more common in children and typically last only a few seconds.
   - Tonic-Clonic Seizures (Grand Mal Seizures): These seizures involve both tonic (stiffening) and clonic (jerking) phases. They can cause loss of consciousness, muscle rigidity, and convulsions, lasting several minutes. Post-seizure confusion and fatigue are common.
   - Myoclonic Seizures: These seizures involve sudden, brief muscle jerks, often affecting both sides of the body. They can occur in clusters and are usually very brief.
   - Atonic Seizures (Drop Attacks): Characterized by a sudden loss of muscle tone, atonic seizures can cause individuals to collapse or fall, posing a risk of injury.
   - Tonic Seizures: These involve a sudden stiffening of muscles, typically lasting less than 20 seconds. They often occur during sleep and can affect both sides of the body.
   - Clonic Seizures: These involve rhythmic, jerking movements of muscles, usually affecting the neck, face, and arms.

3. **Combined Generalized and Focal Epilepsy**
   - Some individuals experience both focal and generalized seizures. This type of epilepsy indicates that abnormal electrical activity can originate in one area of the brain and spread to involve other areas.

4. **Unknown Onset Epilepsy**
   - When the origin of the seizures is not clear, it is classified as unknown onset epilepsy. Over time, as more information is gathered through diagnostic tests and observation, the classification may change.

Types of Seizures

1. **Focal Seizures**
   - Focal Aware Seizures: These seizures do not impair consciousness. Symptoms depend on the area of the brain affected and may include unusual sensations, motor movements, or emotional changes.
   - Focal Impaired Awareness Seizures: These seizures impair consciousness and awareness, often leading to confusion, repetitive movements, or unusual behavior. Individuals may not remember the seizure.

2. **Generalized Seizures**
   - Absence Seizures: Brief episodes of staring or loss of awareness, often accompanied by subtle movements such as eye blinking or lip smacking.
   - Tonic-Clonic Seizures: Characterized by a combination of muscle stiffening (tonic phase) and rhythmic muscle contractions (clonic phase), these seizures often lead to a loss of consciousness and can last several minutes.
   - Myoclonic Seizures: Involve sudden, brief muscle jerks that can affect one or both sides of the body.
   - Atonic Seizures: Sudden loss of muscle tone, causing the individual to fall or drop what they are holding.
   - Tonic Seizures: Sudden stiffening of muscles, often affecting the back, arms, and legs, and typically occurring during sleep.
   - Clonic Seizures: Rhythmic jerking movements of muscles, usually affecting the arms, neck, and face.

3. **Other Seizures**
   - Febrile Seizures: These are typically triggered by fever and are most common in young children. While alarming, they are usually harmless and not indicative of epilepsy.
   - Infantile Spasms: A rare type of epilepsy that occurs in infants, characterized by brief, sudden body stiffening or jerks. It requires prompt medical attention due to potential developmental impacts.

Importance of Accurate Diagnosis

Accurate diagnosis of the type of epilepsy and seizures an individual experiences is crucial for effective treatment and management. Diagnostic tools include:

- Electroencephalogram (EEG): Measures electrical activity in the brain and helps identify abnormal patterns associated with seizures.
- Magnetic Resonance Imaging (MRI): Provides detailed images of the brain to identify structural abnormalities.
- Computerized Tomography (CT) Scan: Offers cross-sectional images of the brain to detect abnormalities.
- Blood Tests: Can help identify underlying conditions that may contribute to seizures.

Causes and Risk Factors

Causes of Epilepsy

Epilepsy can be caused by a wide variety of factors, reflecting its complex nature. It is essential to recognize that in many cases, the exact cause may remain unknown, a situation referred to as idiopathic epilepsy. However, when a cause can be identified, it generally falls into one of the following categories:

1. Genetic Factors
   - Inherited Epilepsy: Some forms of epilepsy are inherited, passed down through families. Genetic epilepsy typically manifests early in life and can sometimes be traced to specific genetic mutations.
   - Genetic Predisposition: Even without a direct hereditary link, some people may have a genetic predisposition to epilepsy, making them more susceptible to seizures when exposed to certain triggers.
2. Structural Brain Abnormalities
   - Congenital Brain Malformations: Developmental issues in the womb can lead to structural abnormalities in the brain, increasing the risk of epilepsy.
   - Tumors and Lesions: Brain tumors or lesions caused by injury or disease can disrupt normal brain activity and lead to seizures.
3. Neurological Diseases and Infections
   - Neurodegenerative Diseases: Conditions such as Alzheimer's disease can damage the brain over time, leading to epilepsy.
   - Infections: Meningitis, encephalitis, and other brain infections can cause inflammation and scarring, resulting in seizures.
4. Head Injuries
   - Traumatic Brain Injury (TBI): Severe head injuries, often from accidents, falls, or sports, can damage brain tissue and lead to epilepsy. The risk is particularly high if the injury penetrates the skull or causes a loss of consciousness.
5. Prenatal and Perinatal Factors
   - Prenatal Brain Injury: Complications during pregnancy, such as inadequate oxygen supply to the brain (hypoxia), infections, or poor maternal nutrition, can lead to epilepsy.
   - Birth Trauma: Difficult or complicated deliveries can sometimes result in brain injuries that increase the risk of developing epilepsy later in life.
6. Metabolic Disorders
   - Imbalance in Brain Chemistry: Conditions that affect the balance of chemicals in the brain, such as hypoglycemia (low blood sugar) or electrolyte imbalances, can cause seizures.
   - Inborn Errors of Metabolism: Rare metabolic disorders present from birth can also lead to epilepsy.

Risk Factors for Epilepsy

While the causes of epilepsy are diverse, several risk factors can increase an individual's likelihood of developing the condition:

1. Age
   - Epilepsy can occur at any age, but it is more common in young children and older adults. The reasons for this vary, with genetic factors often playing a significant role in children and stroke or neurodegenerative diseases being more common in the elderly.
2. Family History
   - Having a family history of epilepsy increases the risk, suggesting a genetic component. This risk is higher if a close relative, such as a parent or sibling, has epilepsy.
3. Medical History
   - Individuals with a history of seizures, particularly febrile seizures (seizures triggered by fever) in childhood, are at an increased risk of developing epilepsy later in life.
   - Previous brain infections, such as meningitis or encephalitis, also elevate the risk.
4. Brain Injuries
   - Sustaining a serious brain injury, particularly one that involves a loss of consciousness or penetration of the skull, significantly increases the risk of developing epilepsy.
5. Stroke and Vascular Diseases
   - Conditions that affect blood flow to the brain, such as stroke or other vascular diseases, can cause brain damage and lead to epilepsy. This is a significant risk factor in older adults.
6. Developmental Disorders
   - Individuals with developmental disorders, such as autism spectrum disorder or neurofibromatosis, have a higher likelihood of having epilepsy.
7. Substance Abuse
   - Chronic alcohol abuse, drug use, and withdrawal from these substances can lead to seizures and increase the risk of epilepsy.
8. Environmental Factors
   - Exposure to certain environmental toxins or chemicals can also elevate the risk, although these cases are less common.

Diagnosis and Medical Assessments for Epilepsy

Diagnosing epilepsy is a multifaceted process that requires a thorough understanding of an individual's medical history, a series of diagnostic tests, and careful observation. The journey to an accurate diagnosis can be both challenging and emotional, as it often involves navigating uncertainties and fears. However, with the right medical support, individuals can find clarity and begin the path to effective management.

Initial Evaluation

The first step in diagnosing epilepsy typically involves a detailed medical evaluation. This initial assessment includes:

1. Medical History
   - Patient's Description: The doctor will ask the patient to describe their seizures in detail. This includes when the seizures started, their frequency, any warning signs, and what happens during and after a seizure.
   - Family History: Information about any family history of epilepsy or other neurological conditions can provide valuable clues.
   - Past Medical History: Details about any previous illnesses, head injuries, infections, or developmental issues are crucial.
2. Witness Accounts
   - Seizure witnesses, often family members or friends, can provide essential observations. They can describe the seizure's appearance, duration, and the patient's behavior before, during, and after the event.
3. Physical and Neurological Examination
   - Physical Examination: The doctor will conduct a general physical exam to check for any signs of underlying conditions that might be causing the seizures.
   - Neurological Examination: This includes assessing motor abilities, sensory function, reflexes, and coordination. It helps identify any neurological abnormalities that might indicate epilepsy.

Diagnostic Tests

To confirm a diagnosis of epilepsy and to understand the underlying causes, several diagnostic tests are employed:

1. Electroencephalogram (EEG)
   - Purpose: An EEG measures electrical activity in the brain. Abnormal brain wave patterns can indicate epilepsy.
   - Procedure: Small electrodes are placed on the scalp to detect electrical activity. The test is painless and typically takes about 20 to 30 minutes, although longer monitoring may be necessary.
   - Video-EEG: In some cases, video monitoring is combined with EEG to correlate seizures with EEG changes.

2. Imaging Tests
  - Magnetic Resonance Imaging (MRI): MRI scans provide detailed images of the brain's structure. They can reveal abnormalities such as tumors, brain damage, or developmental anomalies.
  - Computed Tomography (CT) Scan: A CT scan is used to detect structural changes in the brain, such as bleeding, tumors, or cysts. While less detailed than an MRI, it is quicker and often used in emergency situations.
  - Positron Emission Tomography (PET) and Single-Photon Emission Computed Tomography (SPECT): These imaging techniques help identify areas of the brain with abnormal metabolic activity, often used when surgical treatment is being considered.

3. Blood Tests
  - Purpose: Blood tests can help rule out other conditions that might cause seizures, such as infections, electrolyte imbalances, or metabolic disorders.
  - Genetic Testing: In some cases, genetic testing may be recommended to identify hereditary causes of epilepsy.

4. Neuropsychological Tests
  - These tests assess cognitive functions such as memory, attention, language, and problem-solving skills. They help determine how epilepsy affects brain function and guide treatment planning.

Long-Term Monitoring

In some cases, especially when seizures are infrequent or difficult to diagnose, long-term monitoring may be required:

1. Ambulatory EEG
   - Purpose: Allows for prolonged EEG monitoring while the patient goes about their daily activities.
   - Procedure: The patient wears a portable EEG device that records brain activity over an extended period, typically 24-72 hours.

2. Inpatient Video-EEG Monitoring
   - Purpose: Conducted in a hospital setting, this intensive monitoring allows for the simultaneous recording of seizures and EEG data, providing a comprehensive view of seizure activity.
   - Procedure: Patients are admitted to a specialized epilepsy monitoring unit for continuous video and EEG recording over several days.

Differential Diagnosis

Epilepsy must be differentiated from other conditions that can mimic seizures, such as:

1. Syncope: Fainting or sudden loss of consciousness due to a drop in blood pressure.

2. Migraines: Severe headaches that can sometimes cause neurological symptoms resembling seizures.

3. Psychogenic Non-Epileptic Seizures (PNES): Seizures that have a psychological rather than neurological origin.

4. Sleep Disorders: Conditions like sleep apnea or narcolepsy that can cause abnormal movements or behaviors during sleep.

Conventional Treatments and Their Limitations for Epilepsy

Conventional Treatments

1. Antiepileptic Drugs (AEDs)
   - Overview: AEDs are the most common treatment for epilepsy. They work by stabilizing the electrical activity in the brain to prevent seizures.
   - Types of AEDs:
     - First-Generation AEDs: Includes drugs like phenobarbital, phenytoin (Dilantin), and valproic acid (Depakote). These have been in use for decades.
     - Second-Generation AEDs: Includes drugs like lamotrigine (Lamictal), levetiracetam (Keppra), and topiramate (Topamax). These tend to have fewer side effects and better tolerability.
   - Administration: AEDs can be taken orally, through injections, or via intravenous routes in emergencies.
   - Effectiveness: For about 60-70% of people with epilepsy, AEDs can effectively control seizures.
2. Surgical Interventions
   - Resective Surgery: Involves removing the part of the brain where seizures originate. This is typically considered when seizures are localized and not controlled by medication.
   - Corpus Callosotomy: Involves severing the corpus callosum to prevent the spread of seizures from one hemisphere of the brain to the other. This is usually a last resort.
   - Laser Interstitial Thermal Therapy (LITT): A minimally invasive surgery using lasers to target and destroy the seizure focus.
   - Effectiveness: Surgery can be highly effective for individuals with focal epilepsy, with some achieving complete seizure freedom.
3. Vagus Nerve Stimulation (VNS)
   - Overview: VNS involves implanting a device that sends electrical impulses to the vagus nerve in the neck, which then sends signals to the brain to reduce seizure activity.
   - Procedure: The device is surgically implanted under the skin of the chest, with a wire connecting it to the vagus nerve.
   - Effectiveness: VNS can reduce the frequency and severity of seizures in many patients, though it rarely eliminates them entirely.

4. Ketogenic Diet
   - Overview: A high-fat, low-carbohydrate diet that induces a state of ketosis, which can help control seizures.
   - Administration: The diet must be carefully monitored and adjusted by healthcare professionals.
   - Effectiveness: Particularly effective in children with drug-resistant epilepsy, but also used in adults.

Limitations of Conventional Treatments

1. Side Effects of Antiepileptic Drugs
   - Common Side Effects: Include dizziness, fatigue, weight gain, cognitive impairment, and gastrointestinal issues. These can affect daily functioning and quality of life.
   - Serious Side Effects: Some AEDs carry risks of more severe effects, such as liver toxicity, blood disorders, and severe allergic reactions.
   - Long-Term Effects: Prolonged use of AEDs can lead to bone density loss, hormonal changes, and increased risk of birth defects in pregnant women.
2. Drug Resistance
   - Overview: Approximately 30-40% of people with epilepsy do not achieve seizure control with medication, a condition known as drug-resistant or refractory epilepsy.
   - Implications: This necessitates the exploration of alternative treatments, which may not always be effective or accessible.
3. Surgical Risks
   - Complications: As with any surgery, there are risks involved, including infection, bleeding, and adverse reactions to anesthesia.
   - Cognitive and Behavioral Changes: Brain surgery can sometimes result in cognitive or behavioral changes, depending on the area of the brain involved.
   - Not Suitable for All: Surgery is only an option for a small percentage of epilepsy patients, primarily those with focal seizures.
4. Vagus Nerve Stimulation Limitations
   - Partial Effectiveness: VNS typically reduces the frequency and severity of seizures but rarely results in complete seizure freedom.
   - Side Effects: Can include voice changes, throat pain, shortness of breath, and coughing, particularly during the stimulation period.
5. Challenges of the Ketogenic Diet
   - Strict Regimen: The diet is very restrictive and can be difficult to maintain, particularly for children and families.
   - Nutritional Deficiencies: There is a risk of developing nutritional deficiencies, requiring careful monitoring and supplementation.
   - Side Effects: Common side effects include constipation, high cholesterol, and potential kidney stones.

6. Psychosocial Impact
- Stigma and Isolation: Despite advances in treatment, the social stigma associated with epilepsy can lead to isolation and psychological distress.
- Economic Burden: The cost of long-term treatment, frequent medical appointments, and potential loss of income can be significant.

7. Access to Treatment
- Geographical Barriers: Access to specialized epilepsy care and advanced treatments can be limited in rural or under-resourced areas.
- Healthcare Disparities: Socioeconomic factors can influence the availability and quality of care received by individuals with epilepsy.

Part 2

The Science Behind the Atkins Diet

History of the Atkins Diet

Origins of the Atkins Diet

The story of the Atkins Diet begins with Dr. Robert C. Atkins, a cardiologist who developed the diet in the early 1960s. Dr. Atkins was inspired by a scientific paper published in the Journal of the American Medical Association (JAMA) in 1958 by Dr. Alfred W. Pennington. Pennington's study highlighted the benefits of a low-carbohydrate, high-fat diet for weight loss and metabolic health, challenging the prevailing dietary guidelines of the time. Dr. Atkins decided to experiment with this approach on himself and his patients, observing significant weight loss and improved health markers. Encouraged by these results, he began refining and promoting his dietary regimen.

Publication and Early Reception

In 1972, Dr. Atkins published his first book, "Dr. Atkins' Diet Revolution," which detailed his dietary plan and the science behind it. The book quickly became a bestseller, capturing the public's imagination with its promise of rapid weight loss without the need to count calories or fat grams. The diet's emphasis on protein and fat, while drastically reducing carbohydrates, was revolutionary and counterintuitive to the low-fat, high-carbohydrate dietary recommendations that dominated the era. The initial reception was mixed. While many people reported success with the diet, the medical and nutritional communities were largely skeptical. Critics argued that the diet was unbalanced and potentially harmful, pointing to concerns about high cholesterol levels, heart disease, and other health risks associated with high-fat consumption.

Scientific Scrutiny and Evolution

Throughout the 1980s and 1990s, the Atkins Diet continued to gain popularity, despite ongoing criticism. During this period, Dr. Atkins and his supporters conducted and cited various studies to support the diet's efficacy and safety. Research began to show that low-carbohydrate diets could lead to significant weight loss and improvements in metabolic health, including better blood sugar control and lipid profiles. Dr. Atkins published several revised editions of his book, incorporating new scientific findings and practical advice. These updates helped to refine the diet and address some of the criticisms from the medical community. The most notable of these was "Dr. Atkins' New Diet Revolution," published in 1992, which further solidified the diet's principles and expanded its reach.

Mainstream Acceptance and Popularity

The late 1990s and early 2000s marked a period of widespread acceptance and mainstream popularity for the Atkins Diet. Several factors contributed to this shift:

1. Celebrity Endorsements: High-profile endorsements from celebrities and athletes helped to popularize the diet and increase its credibility.
2. Success Stories: Countless testimonials from individuals who achieved significant weight loss and health improvements fueled public interest and trust in the diet.
3. Scientific Validation: Increasing scientific evidence supported the effectiveness of low-carbohydrate diets, leading to greater acceptance within the medical and nutritional communities.

In 2002, the National Institutes of Health (NIH) sponsored a major study comparing the Atkins Diet to other popular diets. The study found that participants on the Atkins Diet lost more weight and had better improvements in cardiovascular risk factors than those on traditional low-fat diets. This and other studies helped to shift the perception of the Atkins Diet from a fad to a legitimate dietary approach.

Challenges and Controversies

Despite its popularity, the Atkins Diet has faced ongoing challenges and controversies. Critics have continued to raise concerns about the long-term health effects of a high-fat diet, including potential risks for heart disease, kidney function, and bone health. Additionally, the diet's restrictive nature can make it difficult for some individuals to adhere to over the long term. In 2003, Dr. Atkins himself became a point of controversy when he suffered a cardiac arrest and later died from head injuries sustained in a fall. Opponents of the diet seized on this event to question the safety of his dietary recommendations. However, it was later clarified that his heart issues were unrelated to his diet and were instead caused by a chronic viral infection.

The Legacy and Continued Evolution of the Atkins Diet

The Atkins Diet has evolved significantly since its inception. In response to scientific advancements and public feedback, the Atkins Nutritionals company, founded by Dr. Atkins, has continued to refine and update the diet. The modern Atkins Diet includes various phases and allows for a more gradual reintroduction of carbohydrates, making it more flexible and sustainable for a broader audience. Today, the Atkins Diet remains a popular choice for those seeking weight loss and improved metabolic health. It has also inspired numerous other low-carbohydrate diets, such as the ketogenic diet and the paleo diet, which share similar principles.

Key Principles of the Atkins Diet

The Atkins Diet, developed by Dr. Robert C. Atkins in the early 1960s, is renowned for its low-carbohydrate, high-fat approach to weight loss and overall health improvement. Unlike many traditional diets that focus on reducing fat intake, the Atkins Diet centers on carbohydrate restriction to alter the body's metabolism and promote fat burning. The diet is structured around four distinct phases, each with specific guidelines and objectives. Understanding the key principles of the Atkins Diet is crucial for anyone considering this approach to weight management and health.

1. Carbohydrate Restriction

The cornerstone of the Atkins Diet is the significant reduction in carbohydrate intake. By limiting carbs, the diet aims to shift the body's metabolism from burning glucose (derived from carbs) for energy to burning stored fat. This metabolic state is known as ketosis, where the liver produces ketones from fat, which are used as an alternative fuel source.

- Initial Carbohydrate Restriction: In the first phase, the diet restricts carbohydrate intake to about 20 grams per day, primarily from non-starchy vegetables. This drastic reduction helps the body quickly enter ketosis.
- Gradual Increase: As the diet progresses through its phases, carbohydrates are gradually reintroduced in controlled amounts, focusing on high-fiber, nutrient-dense sources.

2. High Fat and Moderate Protein

Contrary to traditional low-fat diets, the Atkins Diet encourages a high intake of fats and moderate consumption of protein. The rationale behind this approach includes:

- Satiety: High-fat and protein-rich foods are more satiating than carbohydrates, helping to reduce overall calorie intake and curb hunger.
- Metabolic Effects: Fats and proteins have different metabolic effects compared to carbohydrates, promoting a more stable blood sugar level and reducing insulin spikes.

3. Controlled Phases

The Atkins Diet is divided into four distinct phases, each with its own goals and guidelines:

1. Induction Phase
   - Duration: Typically lasts two weeks, but can be extended if needed.
   - Objective: To jumpstart weight loss by rapidly inducing ketosis.
   - Guidelines: Carbohydrate intake is limited to 20 grams per day, primarily from non-starchy vegetables. The diet consists mainly of high-fat, moderate-protein foods, such as meat, fish, eggs, cheese, and healthy fats (e.g., avocados, olive oil).

2. Balancing Phase
- Duration: Continues until the individual is within 10 pounds of their target weight.
- Objective: To continue weight loss while reintroducing a wider variety of foods.
- Guidelines: Carbohydrate intake is gradually increased by 5 grams per week. Foods such as nuts, seeds, and berries are reintroduced.

3. Pre-Maintenance Phase
- Duration: Until the individual reaches their goal weight.
- Objective: To find the individual's critical carbohydrate level for maintaining weight.
- Guidelines: Carbohydrate intake is increased by 10 grams per week. The focus is on identifying the maximum amount of carbs one can consume without gaining weight.

4. Lifetime Maintenance Phase
- Duration: Lifelong.
- Objective: To maintain the goal weight and overall health.
- Guidelines: The diet is more flexible but emphasizes the importance of maintaining a low-carbohydrate intake to avoid weight regain. Healthy eating habits and regular monitoring are essential.

4. Focus on Whole, Unprocessed Foods

The Atkins Diet emphasizes the consumption of whole, unprocessed foods. This includes:
- Vegetables: Especially non-starchy ones like leafy greens, broccoli, and bell peppers.
- Proteins: Such as meat, poultry, fish, and eggs.
- Healthy Fats: Including avocados, nuts, seeds, and oils like olive oil and coconut oil.
- Limited Processed Foods: Processed foods, sugary snacks, and refined grains are avoided to minimize empty calories and potential blood sugar spikes.

5. Glycemic Control

One of the key principles of the Atkins Diet is controlling blood sugar levels by avoiding high-glycemic-index (GI) foods that cause rapid spikes in blood sugar. This helps:
- Reduce Cravings: Stable blood sugar levels can help reduce cravings for sugary and high-carb foods.
- Improve Insulin Sensitivity: Lower carbohydrate intake can improve the body's sensitivity to insulin, potentially reducing the risk of type 2 diabetes.

6. Individual Customization

The Atkins Diet is designed to be flexible and customizable based on individual needs and responses. This includes:

- Personalized Carb Levels: As individuals progress through the phases, they identify their own carbohydrate tolerance level to maintain weight and health.
- Adaptation for Special Needs: The diet can be adapted for different lifestyles, dietary preferences, and health conditions.

7. Long-Term Lifestyle Change

Unlike fad diets that often promise quick fixes, the Atkins Diet promotes long-term lifestyle changes. It encourages:

- Sustainable Eating Habits: Focusing on healthy, satisfying foods that can be maintained for life.
- Regular Monitoring: Keeping track of weight, carbohydrate intake, and overall health to make necessary adjustments.

How the Atkins Diet Affects Metabolism

The Atkins Diet, a low-carbohydrate, high-fat dietary regimen, has profound effects on metabolism, fundamentally altering how the body processes and utilizes energy. This shift in metabolic state is central to the diet's effectiveness in promoting weight loss and improving various health markers. Understanding these metabolic changes can help individuals appreciate the scientific principles behind the Atkins Diet and how it can influence their health.

The Role of Carbohydrates in Metabolism

Under typical dietary conditions, carbohydrates are the body's primary source of energy. When consumed, carbohydrates are broken down into glucose, which is then absorbed into the bloodstream. This triggers the release of insulin, a hormone that facilitates the uptake of glucose into cells, where it is used for immediate energy or stored as glycogen in the liver and muscles for later use.

1. Glucose Metabolism:
   - Glucose is the preferred energy source for many tissues and organs, including the brain.
   - Excess glucose can be stored as fat in adipose tissue when glycogen stores are full.
2. Insulin Response:
   - High carbohydrate intake leads to higher insulin levels, which promote glucose uptake and storage.
   - Insulin also inhibits the breakdown of fat, making it harder to lose weight.

Shifting to a Low-Carbohydrate, High-Fat Diet

When carbohydrate intake is drastically reduced, as in the Atkins Diet, the body must adapt to using alternative energy sources. This shift involves several key metabolic changes:

1. Inducing Ketosis:
   - With limited carbohydrates, the body's glycogen stores are quickly depleted.
   - In response, the liver begins to convert fatty acids into ketones, which can be used as an alternative fuel source by many tissues, including the brain.
   - This state is known as ketosis, where ketone bodies (beta-hydroxybutyrate, acetoacetate, and acetone) become the primary energy source.
2. Increased Fat Oxidation:
   - As carbohydrate availability decreases, the body increases the breakdown of stored fat (lipolysis) to meet its energy needs.
   - This leads to an increase in free fatty acids in the bloodstream, which are then transported to the liver for ketone production.

3. Protein Utilization:
   o In the initial phase of the diet, there may be an increase in gluconeogenesis, where amino acids from dietary protein or muscle tissue are converted into glucose.
   o Over time, the body becomes more efficient at utilizing ketones, reducing the need for protein breakdown.

Metabolic Adaptations and Benefits

The metabolic adaptations induced by the Atkins Diet offer several benefits that contribute to weight loss and overall health improvement:

1. Enhanced Fat Burning:
   o The shift to ketosis significantly increases the body's ability to burn fat for fuel.
   o This leads to a reduction in body fat stores, promoting weight loss.
2. Appetite Suppression:
   o Ketones have been shown to have an appetite-suppressing effect, helping to reduce overall calorie intake.
   o High-fat and protein-rich foods are more satiating than carbohydrates, further helping to control hunger.
3. Stable Blood Sugar Levels:
   o Low carbohydrate intake results in fewer blood sugar spikes and a more stable insulin response.
   o This can improve insulin sensitivity and reduce the risk of developing insulin resistance and type 2 diabetes.
4. Improved Lipid Profile:
   o Many individuals on the Atkins Diet experience improvements in their lipid profiles, including increased HDL (good) cholesterol and decreased triglycerides.
   o However, responses can vary, and some individuals may see increases in LDL (bad) cholesterol, necessitating regular monitoring.
5. Increased Energy Levels:
   o Once the body adapts to ketosis, many people report more consistent energy levels and reduced feelings of fatigue.
   o The steady supply of energy from ketones helps prevent the energy crashes associated with fluctuating blood sugar levels.

Potential Challenges and Considerations

While the metabolic effects of the Atkins Diet offer numerous benefits, there are also potential challenges and considerations:

1. Adaptation Period:
   o The initial phase of transitioning to ketosis, often referred to as the "keto flu," can involve symptoms such as fatigue, headache, dizziness, and irritability.
   o These symptoms typically resolve within a few days to a week as the body adapts.

2. Nutrient Intake:
- Reducing carbohydrate intake can limit the consumption of certain nutrient-rich foods, such as fruits, vegetables, and whole grains.
- Careful planning is required to ensure adequate intake of vitamins, minerals, and fiber.

3. Long-Term Sustainability:
- The restrictive nature of the diet can make it challenging for some individuals to maintain over the long term.
- Gradual reintroduction of carbohydrates and finding a balanced approach can help improve adherence.

4. Individual Variability:
- Responses to the Atkins Diet can vary widely among individuals.
- Regular monitoring of health markers, including lipid profiles and kidney function, is essential to ensure the diet is safe and effective.

The Ketogenic Connection: Similarities and Differences

Similarities Between the Atkins and Keto Diets
1. Carbohydrate Restriction
   - Both the Atkins and Keto diets emphasize a significant reduction in carbohydrate intake. This reduction is central to both diets, aiming to shift the body's metabolism from burning glucose to burning fat.
   - Induction Phase (Atkins) and Standard Keto: The initial phase of the Atkins Diet (Induction) restricts carbs to about 20 grams per day, similar to the carbohydrate levels in the standard Keto Diet.
2. Ketosis
   - Both diets aim to induce a state of ketosis, where the body produces ketones from fat to be used as an alternative energy source.
   - Ketone Production: In ketosis, the liver converts fatty acids into ketones, which provide a steady energy supply, especially to the brain and muscles.
3. High Fat Intake
   - Both diets promote high fat intake as the primary source of calories. This is a significant departure from traditional low-fat diets.
   - Healthy Fats: Emphasis is placed on consuming healthy fats such as avocados, nuts, seeds, olive oil, and fatty fish.
4. Moderate Protein Intake
   - Both diets advocate for moderate protein consumption. Excess protein can be converted into glucose through gluconeogenesis, potentially disrupting ketosis.
   - Protein Sources: Common sources include meat, poultry, fish, eggs, and dairy.
5. Weight Loss and Metabolic Benefits
   - Both diets are effective for weight loss and improving various metabolic health markers, including blood sugar control, insulin sensitivity, and lipid profiles.
   - Appetite Suppression: Both diets often result in reduced hunger and appetite, contributing to lower overall calorie intake.

Differences Between the Atkins and Keto Diets
1. Diet Structure and Phases
   o Atkins Diet: The Atkins Diet is divided into four phases:
      i. Induction Phase: Severe carb restriction (20 grams per day) to jumpstart weight loss.
      ii. Balancing Phase: Gradual increase in carb intake (5 grams per week) with continued weight loss.
      iii. Pre-Maintenance Phase: Further increase in carbs (10 grams per week) as weight loss slows.
      iv. Lifetime Maintenance: Maintenance of weight with a sustainable carb level.
   o Keto Diet: The Keto Diet typically does not have structured phases. It maintains a consistent macronutrient ratio focused on high fat (70-80% of calories), moderate protein (15-20%), and very low carbs (5-10%).
2. Flexibility in Carb Intake
   o Atkins Diet: The Atkins Diet allows for a gradual increase in carbohydrate intake through its phases. This provides flexibility for individuals to find their personal carb tolerance while maintaining weight loss and metabolic benefits.
   o Keto Diet: The Keto Diet maintains strict carbohydrate limits throughout, typically around 20-50 grams of net carbs per day, to sustain ketosis.
3. Food Choices and Variety
   o Atkins Diet: The Atkins Diet allows for a broader range of food choices over time, including a gradual reintroduction of higher-carb foods like fruits, whole grains, and legumes in the later phases.
   o Keto Diet: The Keto Diet maintains strict restrictions on high-carb foods, limiting the variety of foods that can be consumed. This includes most fruits, grains, and starchy vegetables.
4. Purpose and Focus
   o Atkins Diet: Primarily designed for weight loss and long-term weight maintenance, with an emphasis on finding a sustainable eating pattern.
   o Keto Diet: Originally developed for therapeutic purposes, particularly for managing epilepsy. It is also used for weight loss, but it emphasizes maintaining a consistent state of ketosis for various health benefits.
5. Scientific Research and Applications
   o Atkins Diet: Supported by research primarily focused on weight loss, metabolic health, and cardiovascular benefits.
   o Keto Diet: Extensive research supports its use not only for weight loss and metabolic health but also for medical conditions like epilepsy, type 2 diabetes, polycystic ovary syndrome (PCOS), and neurodegenerative diseases.

Part 3

Mechanisms of Action: How the Atkins Diet Helps with Epilepsy

The Role of Ketones in Brain Function

Understanding Ketones

Ketones, or ketone bodies, are produced by the liver from fatty acids during periods when glucose availability is low. The primary ketone bodies are:

1. Acetoacetate (AcAc)
2. Beta-hydroxybutyrate (BHB)
3. Acetone

These ketone bodies are transported via the bloodstream to various tissues, including the brain, where they are used as a source of energy.

Energy Metabolism in the Brain

The brain typically relies on glucose as its primary energy source. However, during periods of carbohydrate restriction, prolonged exercise, or starvation, glucose availability can decrease. In such scenarios, ketones become a crucial alternative energy source for the brain:

1. Ketogenesis: When carbohydrate intake is low, insulin levels drop, leading to increased fat breakdown. Fatty acids are converted into ketone bodies in the liver, a process known as ketogenesis.
2. Transport to the Brain: Ketone bodies are transported through the blood-brain barrier via specific transporters (MCT1 and MCT2) that facilitate their uptake into brain cells.
3. Utilization in Neurons: Once inside brain cells, ketone bodies are converted back into acetyl-CoA, which enters the Krebs cycle to produce ATP, the primary energy currency of cells.

Benefits of Ketones for Brain Function

1. Efficient Energy Source
   - Stability: Ketones provide a stable and efficient energy source, reducing fluctuations in energy availability that can occur with glucose metabolism.
   - Efficiency: Ketone metabolism produces more ATP per molecule compared to glucose, providing a more efficient energy yield.

2. Neuroprotection
- Reduced Oxidative Stress: Ketones reduce the production of reactive oxygen species (ROS) during ATP production, thereby lowering oxidative stress and protecting neurons from damage.
- Anti-inflammatory Effects: Ketones have anti-inflammatory properties, which can help reduce neuroinflammation, a factor in many neurological disorders.

3. Cognitive Enhancement
- Mental Clarity: Many individuals report improved mental clarity, focus, and cognitive performance when in ketosis. This is attributed to the brain's efficient utilization of ketones for energy.
- Neurotransmitter Balance: Ketones influence the production of neurotransmitters such as gamma-aminobutyric acid (GABA) and glutamate, promoting a balance that supports cognitive function.

4. Stabilizing Blood Sugar Levels
- Reduced Glycemic Fluctuations: By providing an alternative fuel source, ketones help stabilize blood sugar levels, reducing the risk of hypoglycemia and associated cognitive impairments.

Therapeutic Applications of Ketones in Brain Health

1. Epilepsy
    - Seizure Control: The ketogenic diet has been used for decades to manage epilepsy, particularly in children with drug-resistant forms. Ketones help reduce the frequency and severity of seizures, though the exact mechanisms are not fully understood.

2. Neurodegenerative Diseases
    - Alzheimer's Disease: Research suggests that ketones may improve cognitive function in individuals with Alzheimer's disease by providing an alternative energy source to glucose, which is often impaired in these patients.
    - Parkinson's Disease: Early studies indicate that ketones may have neuroprotective effects that could benefit patients with Parkinson's disease.

3. Traumatic Brain Injury (TBI)
    - Energy Crisis Mitigation: Following a TBI, the brain often experiences an energy crisis due to impaired glucose metabolism. Ketones can provide an alternative energy source, potentially improving recovery outcomes.

4. Mental Health Disorders
    - Mood Stabilization: Emerging evidence suggests that ketogenic diets may help stabilize mood and improve symptoms in conditions such as bipolar disorder and depression. The mechanisms may involve improved energy metabolism and neurotransmitter balance.

5. Cognitive Performance and Aging
    - Cognitive Decline: As the brain ages, its ability to metabolize glucose efficiently can decline, leading to cognitive impairments. Ketones can provide an alternative fuel that supports brain function and may help mitigate age-related cognitive decline.

Potential Risks and Considerations

1. Nutritional Deficiencies
   - Balanced Diet: Adhering to a ketogenic diet requires careful planning to ensure adequate intake of essential nutrients, including vitamins, minerals, and fiber.
2. Ketoacidosis
   - Diabetic Ketoacidosis (DKA): While nutritional ketosis is safe for most individuals, people with type 1 diabetes are at risk of developing diabetic ketoacidosis, a dangerous condition characterized by extremely high levels of ketones.
3. Long-Term Sustainability
   - Adherence: Maintaining a ketogenic diet long-term can be challenging for some individuals due to its restrictive nature. Ensuring variety and palatability in meals is essential for adherence.
4. Medical Supervision
   - Monitoring: Individuals considering a ketogenic diet, especially for therapeutic purposes, should do so under medical supervision to monitor for potential side effects and ensure overall health.

Neuroprotective Effects of Ketones

The neuroprotective effects of ketones are a significant area of interest in neuroscience and nutritional science. Ketones, which are produced during periods of low carbohydrate intake or fasting, provide an alternative energy source to glucose and have been shown to confer various benefits to brain health. These benefits are especially relevant in the context of neurological diseases, cognitive decline, and overall brain function.

Understanding Ketones and Neuroprotection

Ketones, particularly beta-hydroxybutyrate (BHB), acetoacetate (AcAc), and acetone, are produced by the liver from fatty acids during periods of carbohydrate restriction, fasting, or prolonged exercise. These ketones cross the blood-brain barrier and are used by neurons as an efficient energy source. Beyond their role in energy metabolism, ketones exert several neuroprotective effects through various mechanisms:

1. Reduction of Oxidative Stress
2. Anti-Inflammatory Effects
3. Mitochondrial Function Enhancement
4. Excitotoxicity Prevention
5. Gene Expression Modulation

Mechanisms of Neuroprotection

1. Reduction of Oxidative Stress
   - Reactive Oxygen Species (ROS) Reduction: Ketone metabolism produces fewer reactive oxygen species compared to glucose metabolism. This reduction in ROS minimizes oxidative damage to neurons.
   - Antioxidant Enzyme Activation: Ketones upregulate the expression of antioxidant enzymes such as superoxide dismutase (SOD) and catalase, further protecting neurons from oxidative stress.
2. Anti-Inflammatory Effects
   - Inhibition of Pro-Inflammatory Pathways: Ketones inhibit the activity of nuclear factor-kappa B (NF-κB), a key regulator of inflammation. This reduces the production of pro-inflammatory cytokines.
   - Microglial Modulation: Ketones can modulate microglial activation, shifting them from a pro-inflammatory state to a neuroprotective state, thereby reducing neuroinflammation.

3. Mitochondrial Function Enhancement
   - Increased Mitochondrial Efficiency: Ketones improve mitochondrial function by enhancing the efficiency of the electron transport chain, leading to increased ATP production and reduced oxidative stress.
   - Biogenesis Stimulation: Ketones stimulate the production of new mitochondria (mitochondrial biogenesis), enhancing the overall energy capacity of neurons.

4. Excitotoxicity Prevention
   - Glutamate Regulation: Ketones help regulate glutamate levels in the brain. High levels of glutamate can cause excitotoxicity, leading to neuronal damage. Ketones support the conversion of glutamate to gamma-aminobutyric acid (GABA), a calming neurotransmitter.
   - Neuronal Stability: By stabilizing neuronal membranes and reducing excessive neuronal firing, ketones protect against excitotoxic damage.

5. Gene Expression Modulation
   - Epigenetic Effects: Ketones can influence gene expression through epigenetic mechanisms. For instance, BHB acts as a histone deacetylase (HDAC) inhibitor, which can upregulate the expression of genes involved in antioxidant defense and neuronal survival.
   - Neurotrophic Factors: Ketones increase the expression of brain-derived neurotrophic factor (BDNF), a protein that supports the growth, survival, and differentiation of neurons.

Implications for Neurological Conditions

1. Epilepsy
   - Seizure Reduction: The ketogenic diet, which promotes ketone production, has been used for decades to manage epilepsy, particularly in children with drug-resistant forms. Ketones help stabilize neuronal activity and reduce seizure frequency.
   - Long-Term Benefits: Many individuals on a ketogenic diet experience sustained seizure control and improved quality of life.

2. Alzheimer's Disease
   - Glucose Hypometabolism Mitigation: Alzheimer's disease is characterized by impaired glucose metabolism in the brain. Ketones provide an alternative energy source, potentially improving cognitive function.
   - Amyloid Plaque Reduction: Some studies suggest that ketones may reduce the accumulation of amyloid plaques, a hallmark of Alzheimer's pathology.

3. Parkinson's Disease
   - Mitochondrial Support: Parkinson's disease involves mitochondrial dysfunction. Ketones enhance mitochondrial function, which may slow disease progression.
   - Motor Function Improvement: Preliminary research indicates that ketones may improve motor function and reduce symptoms in Parkinson's patients.

4. Traumatic Brain Injury (TBI)
- Energy Crisis Alleviation: Following a TBI, the brain often experiences an energy crisis due to impaired glucose metabolism. Ketones can provide an alternative fuel, potentially aiding in recovery.
- Reduced Inflammation: Ketones' anti-inflammatory properties can mitigate secondary brain injury caused by inflammation.

5. Amyotrophic Lateral Sclerosis (ALS)
- Neuroprotection: ALS involves the progressive loss of motor neurons. Ketones' neuroprotective effects may help slow disease progression and improve patient outcomes.

6. Mental Health Disorders
- Mood Stabilization: Emerging evidence suggests that ketogenic diets may help stabilize mood and improve symptoms in conditions such as bipolar disorder and depression.
- Cognitive Enhancement: By improving mitochondrial function and reducing oxidative stress, ketones may enhance cognitive function and mental clarity.

Practical Considerations and Potential Risks

1. Dietary Implementation
   - Ketogenic Diet: Achieving and maintaining ketosis typically requires adherence to a ketogenic diet, which is high in fats, moderate in protein, and very low in carbohydrates.
   - Monitoring: Regular monitoring of ketone levels can help ensure that the body remains in ketosis, especially for therapeutic purposes.

2. Nutritional Balance
   - Micronutrient Intake: Careful planning is necessary to ensure adequate intake of essential vitamins, minerals, and fiber while following a ketogenic diet.
   - Potential Deficiencies: Individuals may need to supplement with certain nutrients, such as magnesium, potassium, and vitamin D, to prevent deficiencies.

3. Long-Term Sustainability
   - Adherence Challenges: The restrictive nature of a ketogenic diet can be challenging for long-term adherence. Ensuring variety and palatability in meals is essential.
   - Transitioning: Some individuals may choose to transition to a less restrictive low-carbohydrate diet after achieving their health goals.

4. Medical Supervision
   - Individual Variability: Responses to a ketogenic diet can vary widely among individuals. Medical supervision is recommended to monitor for potential side effects and ensure overall health.
   - Specific Conditions: For certain conditions, such as type 1 diabetes, medical guidance is crucial to prevent complications like diabetic ketoacidosis.

Reduction in Seizure Frequency

Historical Context

The use of the ketogenic diet to manage epilepsy dates back to the 1920s when it was first introduced as a treatment for children with intractable seizures. The diet mimics the metabolic state of fasting, during which the body produces ketones from fat as an alternative energy source to glucose. Despite the advent of antiepileptic drugs (AEDs) in the mid-20th century, the ketogenic diet remains a vital option for those who do not respond to medication.

Mechanisms of Action

The ketogenic diet's ability to reduce seizure frequency is attributed to several interconnected mechanisms:

1. Ketone Production and Brain Metabolism
   - Alternative Fuel Source: In the absence of sufficient carbohydrates, the liver converts fatty acids into ketones, which cross the blood-brain barrier and serve as an efficient energy source for neurons.
   - Energy Stability: Ketones provide a stable and sustained energy supply to the brain, preventing the fluctuations in glucose levels that can trigger seizures.
2. Neurotransmitter Balance
   - Glutamate and GABA: The ketogenic diet modulates the balance between excitatory and inhibitory neurotransmitters. It increases the synthesis of gamma-aminobutyric acid (GABA), an inhibitory neurotransmitter, while reducing glutamate, an excitatory neurotransmitter. This balance helps stabilize neuronal activity and prevent seizures.
3. Anti-inflammatory Effects
   - Reduction of Neuroinflammation: Ketones have anti-inflammatory properties that reduce neuroinflammation, a contributing factor to seizure activity. By inhibiting pro-inflammatory pathways, ketones help create a more stable neural environment.
4. Mitochondrial Function
   - Enhanced Mitochondrial Efficiency: The ketogenic diet improves mitochondrial function, leading to increased ATP production and reduced oxidative stress. Enhanced mitochondrial efficiency supports overall brain health and resilience against seizures.
5. Gene Expression Modulation
   - Epigenetic Changes: Ketones can influence gene expression through epigenetic mechanisms. For example, beta-hydroxybutyrate (BHB) acts as a histone deacetylase (HDAC) inhibitor, promoting the expression of genes involved in neuronal protection and stability.

Clinical Applications
1. Pediatric Epilepsy
   o Efficacy: The ketogenic diet has been particularly effective in children with drug-resistant epilepsy. Studies have shown that a significant proportion of children experience a reduction in seizure frequency, with some achieving complete seizure control.
   o Variants: Variations of the ketogenic diet, such as the modified Atkins diet and the low glycemic index treatment (LGIT), have been developed to provide more flexible and sustainable options for children.
2. Adult Epilepsy
   o Growing Evidence: While traditionally used in pediatric cases, increasing evidence supports the ketogenic diet's effectiveness in adults with epilepsy. Adults who do not respond to AEDs have shown significant seizure reduction when adhering to the diet.
3. Specific Epilepsy Syndromes
   o Lennox-Gastaut Syndrome (LGS): The ketogenic diet has been effective in reducing seizures in individuals with LGS, a severe form of epilepsy characterized by multiple types of seizures and intellectual disability.
   o Dravet Syndrome: Patients with Dravet syndrome, a rare and severe form of epilepsy, have also benefited from the ketogenic diet, with many experiencing a substantial decrease in seizure frequency.

Patient Experiences and Case Studies
1. Success Stories
   o Improved Quality of Life: Many patients and families report significant improvements in quality of life following the adoption of the ketogenic diet. Reduced seizure frequency allows for greater independence, better cognitive function, and enhanced overall well-being.
   o Case Studies: Numerous case studies highlight the dramatic impact of the ketogenic diet on seizure control. For example, a study of children with drug-resistant epilepsy found that over 50% experienced a reduction in seizure frequency of more than 50%, and about 10-15% achieved complete seizure freedom.
2. Challenges and Considerations
   o Diet Adherence: Maintaining a strict ketogenic diet can be challenging, particularly in social and family settings. Support from healthcare providers, dietitians, and support groups is crucial for long-term adherence.
   o Side Effects: Some patients may experience side effects, such as gastrointestinal issues, nutrient deficiencies, and changes in lipid profiles. Regular monitoring and adjustments can help manage these side effects.

3. Long-Term Outcomes
- Sustained Benefits: Many patients continue to experience seizure control benefits long-term, even after transitioning to a less restrictive diet. This suggests that the ketogenic diet may induce lasting changes in brain metabolism and function.
- Weaning Off the Diet: In some cases, patients can gradually wean off the ketogenic diet after several years of seizure control, though this should be done under medical supervision to prevent seizure recurrence.

Future Directions and Research

1. Personalized Nutrition
   - Tailored Approaches: Ongoing research aims to personalize the ketogenic diet based on individual metabolic profiles and genetic factors. Tailoring the diet to the specific needs of each patient may enhance its effectiveness and sustainability.
   - Biomarkers: Identifying biomarkers that predict response to the ketogenic diet can help healthcare providers select the most suitable candidates for this therapy.
2. Combination Therapies
   - Integrative Approaches: Combining the ketogenic diet with other treatments, such as new antiepileptic drugs, neurostimulation techniques, and lifestyle interventions, may offer synergistic benefits and further reduce seizure frequency.
3. Broader Applications
   - Other Neurological Disorders: Research continues to explore the ketogenic diet's potential in treating other neurological disorders, such as Alzheimer's disease, Parkinson's disease, and multiple sclerosis. The diet's neuroprotective and anti-inflammatory properties may have broad therapeutic applications.

Part 4

Phases of the Atkins Diet

Induction Phase

Objectives

The Induction Phase of the Atkins Diet is the initial and most restrictive phase, designed to jumpstart weight loss and initiate significant metabolic changes. This phase lays the foundation for the subsequent phases of the diet by shifting the body's metabolism from carbohydrate dependence to fat-burning.

Primary Objectives

1. Initiate Ketosis
   - Carbohydrate Restriction: The primary objective of the Induction Phase is to drastically reduce carbohydrate intake to about 20 grams of net carbs per day. This severe restriction forces the body to deplete its glycogen stores and begin producing ketones from fat for energy.
   - Metabolic Shift: By inducing a state of ketosis, the body shifts its metabolic focus from burning glucose (derived from carbohydrates) to burning stored fat. This metabolic state is essential for achieving rapid weight loss and stabilizing blood sugar levels.

2. Promote Rapid Weight Loss
   - Fat Burning: With the body in ketosis, it becomes highly efficient at burning fat for energy, leading to significant and rapid weight loss. This initial weight loss is often motivating for individuals and helps them commit to the diet.
   - Water Weight: The depletion of glycogen stores also leads to a loss of water weight, as glycogen is stored with water in the body. This initial drop in weight can be quite dramatic and encouraging.

3. Regulate Blood Sugar and Insulin Levels
   - Stabilizing Blood Sugar: The reduction in carbohydrate intake helps stabilize blood sugar levels by minimizing blood sugar spikes and crashes. This stabilization is beneficial for individuals with insulin resistance or type 2 diabetes.
   - Improving Insulin Sensitivity: Lowering carbohydrate intake reduces the need for insulin, which can improve insulin sensitivity and help manage or prevent insulin resistance.

4. Curb Cravings and Appetite
- Reducing Sugar Cravings: By eliminating sugars and refined carbohydrates, the Induction Phase helps reduce cravings for these foods. This change can help individuals break unhealthy eating habits and reduce overall calorie intake.
- Appetite Suppression: The high-fat and moderate-protein content of the diet increases satiety, helping to curb hunger and reduce the desire for frequent snacking.

5. Establish New Eating Habits
- Introduction to Low-Carb Eating: The Induction Phase introduces individuals to the principles of low-carb eating, encouraging the consumption of high-quality proteins, healthy fats, and low-carb vegetables.
- Foundation for Long-Term Success: By adapting to a low-carb lifestyle during the Induction Phase, individuals set the stage for long-term dietary changes that can support sustained weight loss and health improvements.

Secondary Objectives
1. Boost Energy Levels
   - Steady Energy Supply: Once the body adapts to burning fat for fuel, many individuals experience more consistent energy levels throughout the day. This steady energy supply can reduce feelings of fatigue and improve overall well-being.
2. Improve Mental Clarity and Focus
   - Brain Function: Ketones provide a highly efficient energy source for the brain, which can enhance mental clarity, focus, and cognitive performance. Many individuals report improved concentration and reduced brain fog while in ketosis.
3. Reduce Inflammation
   - Anti-Inflammatory Effects: The reduction in carbohydrate intake and the increase in healthy fats can help lower systemic inflammation. This reduction can benefit individuals with inflammatory conditions such as arthritis or metabolic syndrome.
4. Lay the Groundwork for Subsequent Phases
   - Transition to Sustainable Eating: The Induction Phase is designed to be the strictest part of the diet, but it also prepares individuals for the gradual reintroduction of carbohydrates in later phases. This phased approach helps individuals find their personal carbohydrate tolerance while maintaining weight loss and metabolic health.

Practical Considerations

1. Dietary Guidelines
   - Foods to Eat: The Induction Phase emphasizes high-quality proteins (such as meat, poultry, fish, and eggs), healthy fats (such as avocados, olive oil, and nuts), and low-carb vegetables (such as leafy greens, broccoli, and bell peppers).
   - Foods to Avoid: Foods high in carbohydrates, including grains, sugars, starchy vegetables, and most fruits, are restricted. Processed foods and those containing trans fats are also discouraged.
2. Monitoring Progress
   - Tracking Carbohydrate Intake: Keeping track of carbohydrate intake is essential during the Induction Phase to ensure adherence to the 20-gram net carb limit. This can be done using food diaries, apps, or nutrition labels.
   - Measuring Ketone Levels: Some individuals choose to monitor their ketone levels using urine strips, blood meters, or breath analyzers to confirm they are in ketosis.
3. Dealing with Side Effects
   - Keto Flu: Some individuals may experience symptoms such as headache, fatigue, dizziness, and irritability during the first few days of the Induction Phase, commonly referred to as the "keto flu." These symptoms typically resolve within a week as the body adapts to ketosis.
   - Hydration and Electrolytes: Staying well-hydrated and maintaining electrolyte balance (sodium, potassium, and magnesium) can help mitigate side effects and support overall health.

Balancing Phase

Gradual Introduction of Carbs

The Balancing Phase, also known as the Ongoing Weight Loss (OWL) phase, is the second stage of the Atkins Diet. This phase follows the initial Induction Phase and is designed to help individuals continue losing weight while gradually reintroducing carbohydrates into their diet. The gradual introduction of carbs is a crucial aspect of the Balancing Phase, as it helps individuals find their personal carbohydrate tolerance level, maintain steady weight loss, and prepare for the later phases of the diet.

Objectives of the Balancing Phase

1. Continued Weight Loss
   - Steady Progress: The primary goal of the Balancing Phase is to maintain steady, consistent weight loss by gradually increasing carbohydrate intake while staying in a state of ketosis.
   - Avoiding Plateaus: By carefully monitoring carbohydrate intake, individuals can avoid weight loss plateaus and continue making progress toward their goal weight.
2. Identifying Carbohydrate Tolerance
   - Personal Threshold: Each individual has a unique carbohydrate tolerance level, the amount of carbs they can consume while still losing weight. The Balancing Phase helps individuals identify this threshold.
   - Self-Discovery: This process of self-discovery is crucial for long-term success, as it informs dietary choices in the later phases of the Atkins Diet and beyond.
3. Nutritional Balance
   - Variety and Nutrients: The gradual reintroduction of carbs allows for a more varied diet, which can help ensure a balanced intake of essential nutrients, including vitamins, minerals, and fiber.
   - Sustainable Eating Habits: Introducing a wider range of foods helps individuals develop sustainable eating habits that can be maintained for life.

Process of Gradual Carbohydrate Introduction

1. Starting Point
   - Induction Phase Recap: The Balancing Phase begins after completing the Induction Phase, during which carbohydrate intake is limited to about 20 grams of net carbs per day, primarily from non-starchy vegetables.
   - Initial Increase: At the start of the Balancing Phase, individuals typically increase their carbohydrate intake by 5 grams per week, adjusting based on their weight loss progress and ketosis status.

2. Choosing Carbohydrate Sources
- Nutrient-Dense Foods: Emphasis is placed on reintroducing nutrient-dense, high-fiber carbohydrate sources such as low-glycemic fruits, additional vegetables, nuts, and seeds.
- Order of Introduction: The recommended order for reintroducing carbs is:
    a. More non-starchy vegetables (e.g., peppers, broccoli, cauliflower)
    b. Nuts and seeds (e.g., almonds, sunflower seeds)
    c. Berries and other low-glycemic fruits (e.g., strawberries, blueberries)
    d. Full-fat dairy products (e.g., cheese, yogurt)
    e. Legumes (e.g., lentils, black beans)
    f. Whole grains (e.g., quinoa, brown rice) in small amounts as the phase progresses

3. Monitoring and Adjustments
- Weight Tracking: Individuals should monitor their weight regularly to ensure that they are continuing to lose weight at a steady pace. If weight loss stalls, they may need to reduce their carb intake slightly.
- Ketosis Monitoring: Some individuals choose to monitor their ketone levels to ensure they remain in ketosis. This can be done using urine strips, blood meters, or breath analyzers.
- Symptom Observation: Paying attention to how the body responds to reintroduced carbs, including energy levels, cravings, and any gastrointestinal symptoms, is important for making adjustments.

4. Finding the Critical Carbohydrate Level
- Experimentation: The process involves experimentation and careful observation to determine the maximum amount of carbs that can be consumed while still losing weight. This is known as the Critical Carbohydrate Level for Losing (CCLL).
- Incremental Increases: Carbohydrate intake is increased in 5-gram increments each week. If weight loss continues, another 5 grams can be added the following week. If weight loss stalls or reverses, the carb intake is reduced by 5 grams to find a more suitable level.

Practical Tips for the Balancing Phase
1. Meal Planning
    - Diverse Meals: Plan meals that incorporate a variety of the newly introduced carb sources while maintaining a balance of protein, healthy fats, and vegetables.
    - Portion Control: Be mindful of portion sizes, especially when introducing higher-carb foods like nuts, seeds, and fruits.

2. Hydration and Electrolytes
- Staying Hydrated: Drink plenty of water to stay hydrated, especially as carbohydrate intake increases.
- Electrolyte Balance: Ensure adequate intake of electrolytes, such as sodium, potassium, and magnesium, to support overall health and prevent imbalances.

3. Physical Activity
- Exercise Routine: Incorporate regular physical activity to support weight loss, improve metabolic health, and enhance overall well-being.
- Adjusting for Carbs: As carb intake increases, some individuals may find they have more energy for physical activities and can adjust their exercise routines accordingly.

4. Support and Resources
- Educational Materials: Utilize books, websites, and online communities dedicated to the Atkins Diet for recipes, tips, and support.
- Professional Guidance: Consulting with healthcare professionals, such as dietitians or nutritionists, can provide personalized advice and support throughout the Balancing Phase.

Potential Challenges and Solutions

1. Weight Loss Plateaus
   - Identifying Causes: Plateaus can occur due to various factors, including hidden carbs, portion sizes, or insufficient physical activity. Identifying and addressing these factors is crucial.
   - Adjusting Carbs: Reducing carb intake by 5 grams for a week can help overcome a plateau. Additionally, varying macronutrient ratios or incorporating intermittent fasting may be beneficial.

2. Managing Cravings
   - Healthy Alternatives: Address cravings for high-carb foods by finding low-carb alternatives that satisfy the same taste or texture preferences.
   - Mindful Eating: Practice mindful eating techniques to help manage cravings and prevent overeating.

3. Social and Lifestyle Adjustments
   - Social Situations: Navigating social situations and dining out can be challenging. Planning ahead, choosing low-carb options, and communicating dietary needs can help.
   - Long-Term Sustainability: Gradually finding a balance that allows for occasional indulgences while maintaining overall dietary goals is key for long-term success.

Monitoring Seizure Activity

The Balancing Phase of the Atkins Diet is a critical period for individuals with epilepsy who are using the diet as part of their seizure management strategy. During this phase, the gradual reintroduction of carbohydrates necessitates careful monitoring to ensure that any changes in diet do not negatively impact seizure control. Comprehensive monitoring of seizure activity is essential to maintain the therapeutic benefits of the ketogenic state while adjusting to a more varied diet.

Objectives of Monitoring Seizure Activity

1. Maintaining Seizure Control
   - Consistency: Ensuring that the reintroduction of carbohydrates does not lead to an increase in seizure frequency or severity.
   - Early Detection: Identifying any potential triggers or dietary changes that could affect seizure activity.
2. Personalizing the Diet
   - Carbohydrate Threshold: Determining the individual's carbohydrate tolerance level while maintaining seizure control.
   - Adjustments: Making informed adjustments to the diet based on seizure activity and overall health.
3. Overall Health and Well-being
   - Nutritional Balance: Ensuring that the diet remains nutritionally balanced while increasing carbohydrate intake.
   - Long-term Management: Developing sustainable dietary habits that support both seizure control and overall health.

Methods of Monitoring Seizure Activity

1. Seizure Diaries and Logs
   - Daily Recording: Keeping a detailed daily log of seizure activity, including the date, time, duration, and characteristics of each seizure.
   - Triggers and Patterns: Documenting potential triggers, such as specific foods, stress, sleep patterns, or other environmental factors. This helps identify any correlations between dietary changes and seizure activity.
2. Carbohydrate Tracking
   - Net Carb Counting: Monitoring the intake of net carbohydrates (total carbs minus fiber) to ensure adherence to the prescribed carb limits during the Balancing Phase.
   - Incremental Increases: Gradually increasing carbohydrate intake by 5 grams per week and observing any changes in seizure activity.

3. Ketone Monitoring
- Blood Ketone Meters: Using blood ketone meters to measure beta-hydroxybutyrate (BHB) levels, providing accurate data on the body's state of ketosis.
- Urine or Breath Tests: Utilizing urine strips or breath analyzers as less invasive methods to monitor ketone levels, although these may be less precise than blood measurements.

4. Regular Medical Check-ups
- Neurological Assessments: Scheduling regular appointments with a neurologist or epilepsy specialist to review seizure activity and make necessary adjustments to the diet or medication.
- Nutritional Evaluations: Consulting with a dietitian or nutritionist to ensure the diet remains balanced and to address any nutritional deficiencies.

5. Technology and Apps
- Seizure Tracking Apps: Utilizing mobile apps designed to track seizure activity, medication, diet, and other health metrics. These apps can provide detailed reports and trends for healthcare providers.
- Wearable Devices: Exploring wearable devices that can detect and log seizures, offering additional data and insights into seizure patterns.

Practical Considerations
1. Dietary Adjustments
    - Slow Reintroduction: Reintroduce carbohydrates slowly and monitor for any changes in seizure activity. If seizures increase, reduce carbohydrate intake and consult with a healthcare provider.
    - Food Quality: Focus on reintroducing high-quality, nutrient-dense carbohydrates such as low-glycemic fruits, vegetables, nuts, and seeds.
2. Consistency in Monitoring
    - Routine Tracking: Consistently track seizure activity and dietary intake to identify patterns and make informed adjustments.
    - Detailed Documentation: Maintain detailed records, including the type and amount of foods consumed, to help pinpoint any potential dietary triggers.
3. Communication with Healthcare Providers
    - Regular Updates: Provide regular updates to healthcare providers about seizure activity and dietary changes. Collaborative management is essential for effective seizure control.
    - Emergency Plans: Have a plan in place for managing breakthrough seizures, including when to seek emergency medical help.

Addressing Potential Challenges

1. Plateaus and Increases in Seizures
   - Identifying Triggers: Work with healthcare providers to identify potential triggers if seizures increase during the Balancing Phase.
   - Adjusting Carbs: Temporarily reduce carbohydrate intake if an increase in seizures is observed. Gradually reintroduce carbs again under medical supervision.
2. Managing Side Effects
   - Nutrient Deficiencies: Monitor for signs of nutrient deficiencies, such as fatigue, muscle cramps, or skin issues. Supplement the diet with vitamins and minerals if needed.
   - Gastrointestinal Issues: Address any gastrointestinal issues that arise with dietary changes by adjusting fiber intake and staying hydrated.
3. Emotional and Psychological Support
   - Stress Management: Recognize that stress and anxiety can impact seizure control. Incorporate stress-reducing activities such as yoga, meditation, or counseling.
   - Support Groups: Engage with support groups or online communities for individuals with epilepsy and those following the ketogenic diet. Sharing experiences and advice can provide valuable support and motivation.

Adjusting Macronutrient Ratios

The Balancing Phase of the Atkins Diet is a critical period of adjustment and fine-tuning. During this phase, individuals gradually reintroduce carbohydrates into their diet while continuing to lose weight and maintain metabolic health. A key aspect of this phase is adjusting macronutrient ratios—specifically the proportions of carbohydrates, fats, and proteins—to ensure ongoing weight loss, nutritional balance, and overall well-being.

Objectives of Adjusting Macronutrient Ratios

1. Continued Weight Loss
   - Steady Progress: Adjusting macronutrient ratios helps maintain a caloric deficit and promotes steady, consistent weight loss.
   - Avoiding Plateaus: By fine-tuning macronutrient intake, individuals can prevent or overcome weight loss plateaus.
2. Maintaining Ketosis
   - Ketone Production: Ensuring that carbohydrate intake remains low enough to sustain ketone production and maintain a state of ketosis.
   - Energy Efficiency: Using ketones as a primary energy source enhances metabolic efficiency and supports weight loss.
3. Nutritional Balance
   - Essential Nutrients: Adjusting macronutrient ratios to include a variety of nutrient-dense foods that provide essential vitamins, minerals, and fiber.
   - Diet Diversity: Gradually introducing a wider range of foods to promote a balanced and sustainable diet.
4. Personalization and Sustainability
   - Individual Needs: Tailoring macronutrient ratios to individual metabolic responses, preferences, and lifestyle factors.
   - Long-Term Adherence: Developing a sustainable eating pattern that can be maintained beyond the Balancing Phase.

Strategies for Adjusting Macronutrient Ratios

1. Carbohydrate Reintroduction
   - Incremental Increases: Begin with a low carbohydrate intake (about 20 grams per day) from the Induction Phase and gradually increase by 5 grams per week.
   - High-Fiber Carbs: Focus on reintroducing high-fiber, nutrient-dense carbohydrates such as non-starchy vegetables, nuts, seeds, and low-glycemic fruits.
   - Monitoring Response: Carefully monitor weight, ketone levels, and overall well-being with each increase in carbohydrate intake to determine the appropriate amount.

2. Protein Management
- Moderate Intake: Maintain a moderate protein intake to support muscle mass and overall health without disrupting ketosis.
- Quality Sources: Choose high-quality protein sources such as lean meats, poultry, fish, eggs, and plant-based options like tofu and legumes.
- Balancing Act: Ensure protein intake is sufficient to meet daily requirements but not excessive, as excess protein can be converted into glucose through gluconeogenesis.

3. Fat Consumption
- Primary Energy Source: Continue to rely on healthy fats as the primary source of energy, especially while carbohydrate intake remains low.
- Variety of Fats: Incorporate a variety of healthy fats, including monounsaturated fats (olive oil, avocados), polyunsaturated fats (nuts, seeds, fatty fish), and saturated fats (coconut oil, butter) in moderation.
- Satiety and Taste: Use fats to enhance the flavor and satiety of meals, helping to reduce hunger and maintain a caloric deficit.

4. Macronutrient Ratios
- Starting Ratios: During the early Balancing Phase, a common macronutrient ratio is approximately 60-70% fat, 20-30% protein, and 5-10% carbohydrates.
- Adjusting Ratios: As carbohydrate intake increases, adjust the ratios to maintain weight loss and ketosis. This may involve slightly reducing fat intake while keeping protein intake consistent.
- Personalization: Individualize the ratios based on metabolic response, activity level, and personal preferences to ensure long-term adherence and success.

Practical Considerations
1. Meal Planning and Preparation
   - Balanced Meals: Plan meals that incorporate the adjusted macronutrient ratios, ensuring each meal includes a balance of fats, proteins, and gradually increasing carbohydrates.
   - Portion Control: Be mindful of portion sizes to manage caloric intake and maintain the desired macronutrient balance.
2. Tracking and Monitoring
   - Food Diaries: Keep a detailed food diary to track macronutrient intake, weight, ketone levels, and any changes in health or well-being.
   - Regular Check-ins: Schedule regular check-ins with healthcare providers or dietitians to review progress and make necessary adjustments.

3. Addressing Plateaus and Challenges
- Identifying Issues: If weight loss stalls or other issues arise, review dietary intake, physical activity, and lifestyle factors to identify potential causes.
- Making Adjustments: Adjust macronutrient ratios, meal timing, or caloric intake to overcome plateaus and continue making progress.

4. Physical Activity
- Incorporate Exercise: Engage in regular physical activity to support weight loss, improve metabolic health, and enhance overall well-being.
- Adjusting for Activity: Adjust macronutrient intake based on activity level, ensuring adequate energy and recovery support.

Potential Challenges and Solutions

1. Balancing Macronutrients
   - Finding the Right Balance: It can be challenging to find the right balance of macronutrients that supports weight loss and ketosis while meeting nutritional needs. Experimenting and adjusting based on feedback is key.
   - Professional Guidance: Working with a dietitian or nutritionist can provide personalized guidance and help fine-tune macronutrient ratios.

2. Maintaining Ketosis
   - Carb Tolerance: Each individual's carbohydrate tolerance level varies. Monitoring ketone levels and adjusting carbohydrate intake accordingly is essential to maintain ketosis.
   - Hidden Carbs: Be vigilant about hidden carbs in processed foods, sauces, and condiments that could disrupt ketosis.

3. Nutritional Deficiencies
   - Micronutrient Intake: Ensure adequate intake of vitamins and minerals through a varied diet and, if necessary, supplements. Focus on nutrient-dense foods like leafy greens, nuts, seeds, and low-glycemic fruits.
   - Fiber Intake: Reintroduce high-fiber carbohydrates gradually to support digestive health and prevent constipation.

Pre-Maintenance Phase

Stabilizing Ketosis

The Pre-Maintenance Phase of the Atkins Diet is a transitional stage where the focus shifts from ongoing weight loss to establishing a sustainable eating pattern that will maintain your target weight and health goals. One of the key objectives during this phase is stabilizing ketosis, ensuring that the body continues to use fat as its primary energy source while allowing for a more flexible and varied diet.

Objectives of Stabilizing Ketosis

1. Maintain Weight Loss
   - Preventing Weight Regain: Ensuring that the body remains in a state of ketosis helps prevent weight regain as carbohydrate intake is gradually increased.
   - Steady Transition: Stabilizing ketosis provides a steady metabolic environment, making the transition to a maintenance diet smoother and more sustainable.
2. Optimize Metabolic Health
   - Insulin Sensitivity: Maintaining ketosis supports improved insulin sensitivity, reducing the risk of metabolic disorders such as type 2 diabetes.
   - Stable Blood Sugar Levels: A ketogenic state helps stabilize blood sugar levels, minimizing fluctuations that can lead to cravings and overeating.
3. Establish Long-Term Eating Habits
   - Balanced Diet: Gradually increasing carbohydrate intake while maintaining ketosis encourages the development of balanced and sustainable eating habits.
   - Personalized Nutrition: Identifying individual carbohydrate tolerance levels ensures that the diet can be personalized to support long-term health and weight maintenance.

Strategies for Stabilizing Ketosis

1. Gradual Carbohydrate Increase
   - Incremental Adjustments: Continue to increase carbohydrate intake in small increments, typically by 10 grams per week. This cautious approach helps identify the maximum amount of carbs that can be consumed without disrupting ketosis.
   - Monitor Response: Carefully monitor weight, ketone levels, and overall well-being with each increase in carbohydrate intake. If ketone levels drop or weight begins to increase, reduce carbohydrate intake slightly.

2. Choosing the Right Carbohydrates
- Low-Glycemic Foods: Focus on reintroducing low-glycemic carbohydrates that have a minimal impact on blood sugar levels. These include non-starchy vegetables, berries, nuts, seeds, and legumes.
- Nutrient-Dense Options: Select nutrient-dense carbohydrates that provide essential vitamins, minerals, and fiber, supporting overall health and digestive function.

3. Balancing Macronutrients
- Consistent Fat Intake: Maintain a high intake of healthy fats to ensure that fat remains the primary energy source. Include a variety of fats such as avocados, olive oil, nuts, seeds, and fatty fish.
- Moderate Protein: Keep protein intake at a moderate level to support muscle maintenance and overall health. Avoid excessive protein consumption, as it can lead to gluconeogenesis, which may interfere with ketosis.

4. Monitoring Ketone Levels
- Regular Testing: Use blood ketone meters, urine strips, or breath analyzers to regularly monitor ketone levels. This helps ensure that the body remains in a state of ketosis as carbohydrate intake increases.
- Adjusting Intake: If ketone levels drop, reduce carbohydrate intake or increase fat consumption to restore and stabilize ketosis.

5. Consistent Meal Timing
- Regular Meals: Eating regular meals at consistent times helps stabilize blood sugar levels and supports the body's metabolic rhythms.
- Avoiding Fasting: While intermittent fasting can be beneficial for some, it may not be necessary during the Pre-Maintenance Phase. Focus on balanced meals that provide steady energy throughout the day.

Identifying Personal Carb Threshold

The Pre-Maintenance Phase of the Atkins Diet marks a pivotal stage where individuals fine-tune their carbohydrate intake to establish a sustainable, long-term eating plan. A key goal during this phase is identifying your personal carbohydrate threshold—the maximum amount of carbohydrates you can consume while maintaining weight and metabolic health without triggering weight gain or reverting to poor metabolic markers. This comprehensive discussion explores the significance, methods, and practical considerations involved in identifying your personal carbohydrate threshold.

Importance of Identifying Personal Carb Threshold

1. Weight Maintenance
   - Preventing Regain: Understanding your carb threshold helps maintain your target weight by preventing excessive carbohydrate intake that could lead to weight regain.
   - Sustainable Eating: Establishing a clear carb threshold allows for a more flexible and sustainable diet that supports long-term weight management.
2. Metabolic Health
   - Blood Sugar Control: Identifying the right amount of carbohydrates helps maintain stable blood sugar levels, reducing the risk of insulin resistance and type 2 diabetes.
   - Ketosis Management: Determining your carb threshold ensures that you stay within a range that supports ketosis, if desired, or maintains overall metabolic health.
3. Personalization and Flexibility
   - Tailored Diet: Personalizing your carbohydrate intake based on your individual metabolic response allows for a more enjoyable and diverse diet.
   - Long-Term Success: A personalized approach to carbohydrate consumption enhances long-term adherence and success in maintaining health goals.

Methods for Identifying Personal Carb Threshold

1. Incremental Carb Increases
   - Gradual Introduction: Start by gradually increasing your carbohydrate intake from the level established during the Induction and Balancing Phases. Typically, this involves adding 10 grams of net carbs per week.
   - Monitor and Adjust: Carefully monitor your weight, ketone levels (if maintaining ketosis), and overall well-being with each incremental increase. Adjust the intake based on your body's response.

2. Tracking and Monitoring
- Food Diary: Keep a detailed food diary to track your daily carbohydrate intake, noting the type and amount of carbs consumed, as well as any changes in weight, energy levels, and health markers.
- Weight Monitoring: Regularly monitor your weight to detect any changes. A stable weight indicates that you are within your carbohydrate threshold, while weight gain suggests that you may have exceeded it.
- Ketone Testing: If you aim to stay in ketosis, use ketone meters, urine strips, or breath analyzers to monitor ketone levels. Adjust carbohydrate intake based on ketone readings to maintain ketosis.

3. Glycemic Response Monitoring
- Blood Glucose Testing: Use a blood glucose meter to check your blood sugar levels before and after meals. This helps identify how different carbohydrates affect your blood sugar levels and can guide adjustments to your carb intake.
- Continuous Glucose Monitors (CGMs): For more detailed data, consider using a CGM, which provides continuous blood sugar readings and helps identify patterns and responses to various foods.

4. Symptoms and Well-being
- Energy Levels: Pay attention to your energy levels and overall well-being. A sudden drop in energy or feelings of fatigue may indicate that you have exceeded your carbohydrate threshold.
- Digestive Health: Monitor digestive symptoms, as increased carbohydrate intake can affect gut health. Bloating, gas, or other digestive issues may suggest the need for adjustments.

Practical Considerations
1. Choosing Carbohydrate Sources
   - Low-Glycemic Options: Focus on low-glycemic carbohydrates that have a minimal impact on blood sugar levels, such as non-starchy vegetables, berries, nuts, seeds, and legumes.
   - Nutrient-Dense Foods: Select nutrient-dense carbohydrates that provide essential vitamins, minerals, and fiber. This supports overall health and helps prevent nutrient deficiencies.
2. Meal Planning and Preparation
   - Balanced Meals: Plan meals that include a balance of proteins, healthy fats, and gradually increasing amounts of carbohydrates. This helps maintain satiety and supports overall nutritional balance.
   - Portion Control: Be mindful of portion sizes to manage caloric intake and maintain the desired macronutrient balance.

3. Physical Activity
- Exercise Routine: Engage in regular physical activity to support metabolic health and weight maintenance. Exercise can also increase your carbohydrate tolerance by improving insulin sensitivity.
- Adjusting Intake: Adjust your carbohydrate intake based on your activity level, ensuring that you have adequate energy for exercise and recovery.

4. Hydration and Electrolytes
- Stay Hydrated: Drink plenty of water to stay hydrated, especially as carbohydrate intake increases. Proper hydration supports overall health and helps prevent dehydration-related side effects.
- Electrolyte Balance: Ensure adequate intake of electrolytes, such as sodium, potassium, and magnesium, to support metabolic function and prevent imbalances.

Addressing Potential Challenges
1. Weight Fluctuations
   - Identifying Causes: If you experience weight gain, review your dietary intake, physical activity, and lifestyle factors to identify potential causes.
   - Making Adjustments: Reduce carbohydrate intake by 10 grams per week until weight stabilizes. Reassess and adjust as needed to find your carb threshold.
2. Maintaining Ketosis
   - Carb Tolerance: Each individual's carbohydrate tolerance level varies. Monitoring ketone levels and adjusting carbohydrate intake accordingly is essential to maintain ketosis.
   - Hidden Carbs: Be vigilant about hidden carbs in processed foods, sauces, and condiments that could disrupt ketosis.
3. Managing Cravings and Hunger
   - Healthy Alternatives: Address cravings for high-carb foods by finding low-carb alternatives that satisfy the same taste or texture preferences.
   - Mindful Eating: Practice mindful eating techniques to help manage cravings and prevent overeating.

Breakfast Recipes

1. Egg and Avocado Salad

Ingredients:

- 4 large eggs
- 2 ripe avocados
- 2 tablespoons mayonnaise (preferably made with avocado oil)
- 1 tablespoon lemon juice
- 1 teaspoon Dijon mustard
- 1 tablespoon chopped fresh chives
- 1 tablespoon chopped fresh parsley
- 1 tablespoon olive oil
- 1 teaspoon smoked paprika
- Freshly ground black pepper, to taste

Instructions:

1. Place the eggs in a saucepan and cover with cold water. Bring to a boil over medium-high heat. Once boiling, cover the saucepan, remove from heat, and let stand for 10-12 minutes.
2. Drain the hot water and transfer the eggs to a bowl of ice water to cool. Once cool, peel the eggs and chop them into small pieces.
3. In a large mixing bowl, combine the mayonnaise, lemon juice, Dijon mustard, olive oil, smoked paprika, and black pepper. Mix well to combine.
4. Add the chopped eggs to the bowl and gently fold them into the mayonnaise mixture.
5. Cut the avocados in half, remove the pits, and dice the flesh. Add the diced avocados to the egg mixture and gently mix to combine.
6. Sprinkle with chopped chives and parsley.
7. Serve immediately, or chill in the refrigerator for up to 2 hours before serving.

Nutrition Info Per Serving (1 serving):

- Calories: 320
- Total Fat: 28g
- Saturated Fat: 4g
- Cholesterol: 215mg
- Sodium: 150mg
- Total Carbohydrates: 6g
- Dietary Fiber: 4g
- Sugars: 1g
- Protein: 10g

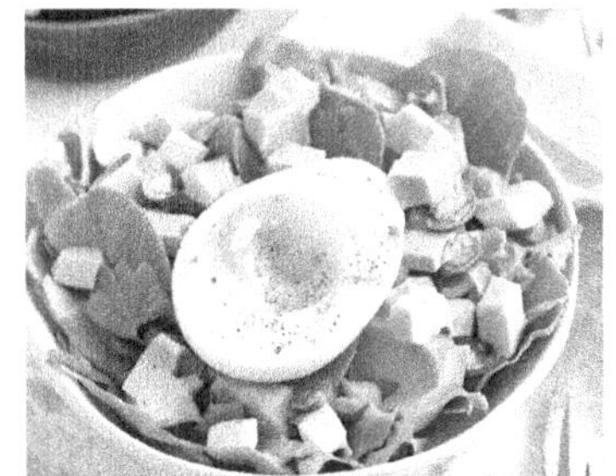

Number of Servings: 4 Cooking Time: 20 minutes (plus 10-12 minutes for egg cooking)

2. Spinach and Mushroom Omelette

Ingredients:

- 3 large eggs
- 1/2 cup fresh spinach, chopped
- 1/2 cup mushrooms, sliced
- 1/4 cup heavy cream
- 1/4 cup grated cheddar cheese
- 2 tablespoons butter
- 1/2 teaspoon garlic powder
- Freshly ground black pepper, to taste

Instructions:

1. In a medium mixing bowl, whisk together the eggs, heavy cream, garlic powder, and black pepper until well combined.
2. Heat 1 tablespoon of butter in a non-stick skillet over medium heat. Add the mushrooms and cook until they are soft and have released their moisture, about 5 minutes.
3. Add the chopped spinach to the skillet and cook until wilted, about 2 minutes. Remove the mushrooms and spinach from the skillet and set aside.
4. Add the remaining tablespoon of butter to the skillet and pour in the egg mixture. Cook until the edges start to set, about 2 minutes.
5. Sprinkle the cheddar cheese evenly over the eggs, then add the cooked mushrooms and spinach on one half of the omelette.
6. Carefully fold the omelette in half and continue to cook until the cheese is melted and the eggs are fully set, about 2-3 more minutes.
7. Slide the omelette onto a plate and serve immediately.

Nutrition Info Per Serving (1 serving):

- Calories: 420
- Total Fat: 37g
- Saturated Fat: 20g
- Cholesterol: 345mg
- Sodium: 280mg
- Total Carbohydrates: 5g
- Dietary Fiber: 1g
- Sugars: 2g
- Protein: 17g

Number of Servings: 1 Cooking Time: 15 minutes

3. Cheese and Herb Frittata

Ingredients:

- 6 large eggs
- 1/2 cup heavy cream
- 1 cup shredded mozzarella cheese
- 1/4 cup grated Parmesan cheese
- 1/4 cup chopped fresh basil
- 1/4 cup chopped fresh parsley
- 2 tablespoons olive oil
- 1/2 teaspoon garlic powder
- Freshly ground black pepper, to taste

Instructions:

1. Preheat your oven to 350°F (175°C).
2. In a large mixing bowl, whisk together the eggs, heavy cream, garlic powder, and black pepper until well combined.
3. Stir in the mozzarella cheese, Parmesan cheese, basil, and parsley.
4. Heat the olive oil in an oven-safe skillet over medium heat. Pour the egg mixture into the skillet and cook until the edges start to set, about 3-4 minutes.
5. Transfer the skillet to the preheated oven and bake until the frittata is fully set and golden on top, about 15-20 minutes.
6. Remove the skillet from the oven and let the frittata cool for a few minutes before slicing and serving.

Nutrition Info Per Serving (1 serving):

- Calories: 340
- Total Fat: 30g
- Saturated Fat: 16g
- Cholesterol: 245mg
- Sodium: 300mg
- Total Carbohydrates: 3g
- Dietary Fiber: 0.5g
- Sugars: 1g
- Protein: 16g

Number of Servings: 4

Cooking Time: 25-30 minutes

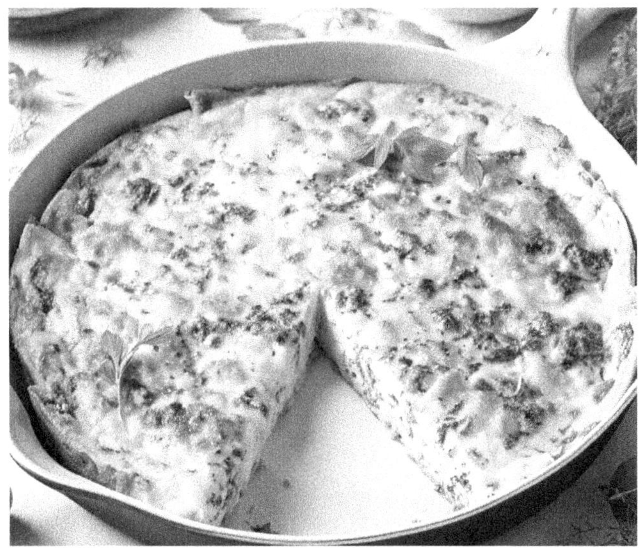

4. Bacon and Egg Cups

Ingredients:

- 8 slices of bacon
- 8 large eggs
- 1/2 cup shredded cheddar cheese
- 1/4 cup heavy cream
- 1/4 cup chopped chives
- 1/2 teaspoon smoked paprika

Instructions:

1. Preheat your oven to 375°F (190°C).
2. Lightly grease a muffin tin with butter or cooking spray.
3. Line each muffin cup with a slice of bacon, forming a cup shape.
4. In a mixing bowl, whisk together the eggs, heavy cream, smoked paprika, and chives.
5. Pour the egg mixture into each bacon-lined cup, filling about three-quarters full.
6. Sprinkle shredded cheddar cheese on top of each cup.
7. Bake in the preheated oven for 15-20 minutes, or until the eggs are set and the bacon is crispy.
8. Allow to cool slightly before serving.

Nutrition Info Per Serving (1 cup):

- Calories: 210
- Total Fat: 17g
- Saturated Fat: 7g
- Cholesterol: 215mg
- Sodium: 320mg
- Total Carbohydrates: 1g
- Dietary Fiber: 0g
- Sugars: 0g
- Protein: 13g

Number of Servings: 8
Cooking Time: 20 minutes

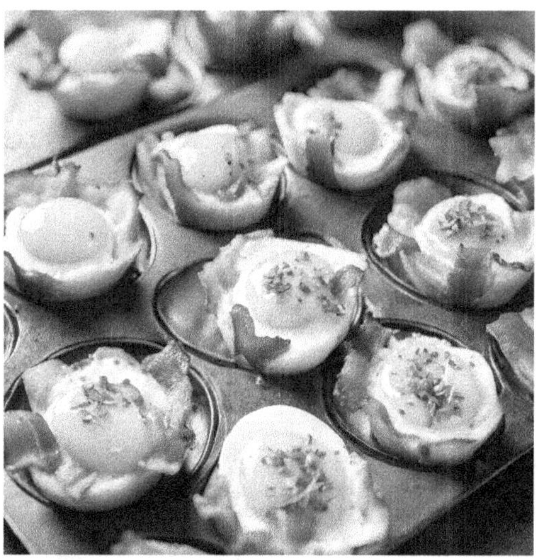

5. Sausage and Pepper Skillet

Ingredients:

- 1 lb Italian sausage (preferably without added sugar)
- 1 red bell pepper, sliced
- 1 yellow bell pepper, sliced
- 1 green bell pepper, sliced
- 1 small onion, sliced
- 1/4 cup olive oil
- 2 cloves garlic, minced
- 1 teaspoon dried oregano
- 1 teaspoon dried basil
- 1/2 teaspoon smoked paprika

Instructions:

1. Heat olive oil in a large skillet over medium-high heat.
2. Add the sausage and cook until browned, about 5-7 minutes. Remove sausage from skillet and set aside.
3. In the same skillet, add the sliced bell peppers, onion, and garlic. Sauté until the vegetables are tender, about 5-7 minutes.
4. Return the sausage to the skillet and add the oregano, basil, and smoked paprika. Stir to combine.
5. Cook for an additional 3-5 minutes, until the sausage is fully cooked and the flavors are well combined.
6. Serve hot.

Nutrition Info Per Serving (1 serving):

- Calories: 320
- Total Fat: 26g
- Saturated Fat: 8g
- Cholesterol: 70mg
- Sodium: 620mg
- Total Carbohydrates: 5g
- Dietary Fiber: 1g
- Sugars: 2g
- Protein: 15g

Number of Servings: 4
Cooking Time: 20 minutes

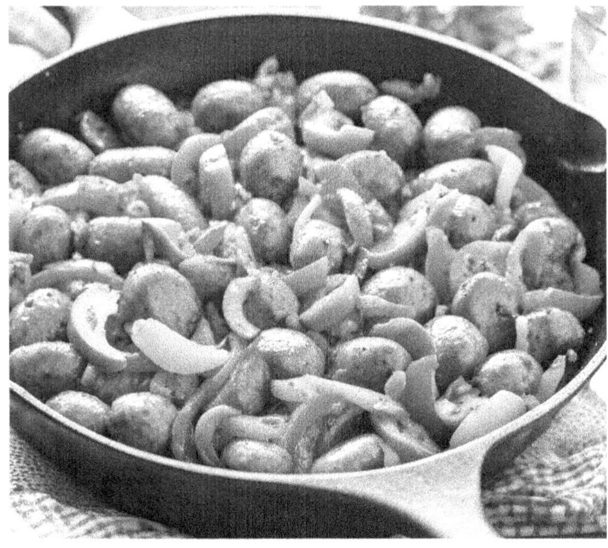

6. Chia Pudding with Coconut Milk

Ingredients:

- 1 cup full-fat coconut milk
- 1/4 cup chia seeds
- 1 teaspoon vanilla extract
- 2 tablespoons shredded unsweetened coconut
- 1 tablespoon chopped almonds
- 1 tablespoon sugar-free sweetener (optional)

Instructions:

1. In a mixing bowl, combine the coconut milk, chia seeds, vanilla extract, and sugar-free sweetener (if using). Stir well to combine.
2. Cover and refrigerate for at least 4 hours or overnight, allowing the chia seeds to absorb the liquid and thicken.
3. Before serving, stir the pudding to break up any clumps.
4. Top with shredded coconut and chopped almonds.
5. Serve chilled.

Nutrition Info Per Serving (1 serving):

- Calories: 240
- Total Fat: 20g
- Saturated Fat: 15g
- Cholesterol: 0mg
- Sodium: 10mg
- Total Carbohydrates: 9g
- Dietary Fiber: 7g
- Sugars: 1g
- Protein: 4g

Number of Servings: 2

Cooking Time: 10 minutes (plus 4 hours chilling time)

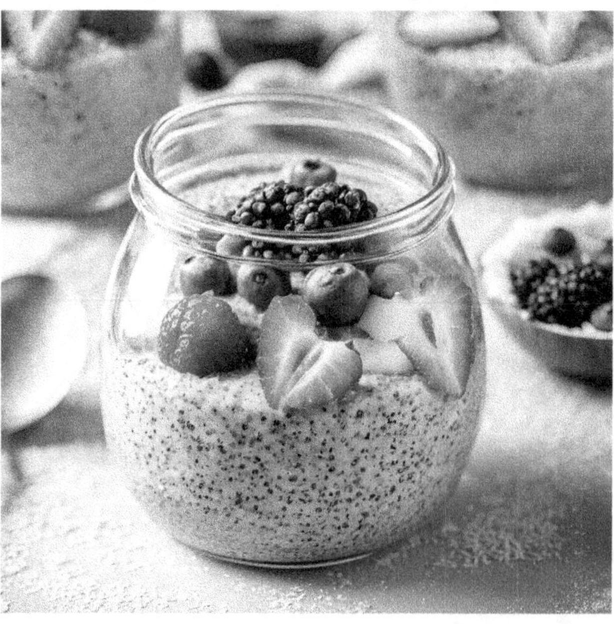

7. Zucchini and Parmesan Bake

Ingredients:

- 2 medium zucchinis, thinly sliced
- 1 cup grated Parmesan cheese
- 1/2 cup heavy cream
- 1/4 cup chopped fresh basil
- 2 cloves garlic, minced
- 2 tablespoons olive oil
- 1 teaspoon dried oregano

Instructions:

1. Preheat your oven to 375°F (190°C).
2. Grease a baking dish with olive oil.
3. Layer the zucchini slices in the baking dish.
4. In a mixing bowl, combine the heavy cream, minced garlic, oregano, and half of the Parmesan cheese. Mix well.
5. Pour the cream mixture over the zucchini slices.
6. Sprinkle the remaining Parmesan cheese on top.
7. Bake in the preheated oven for 25-30 minutes, or until the zucchini is tender and the cheese is golden and bubbly.
8. Garnish with chopped fresh basil before serving.

Nutrition Info Per Serving (1 serving):

- Calories: 210
- Total Fat: 18g
- Saturated Fat: 9g
- Cholesterol: 45mg
- Sodium: 270mg
- Total Carbohydrates: 5g
- Dietary Fiber: 2g
- Sugars: 2g
- Protein: 8g

Number of Servings: 4
Cooking Time: 30 minutes

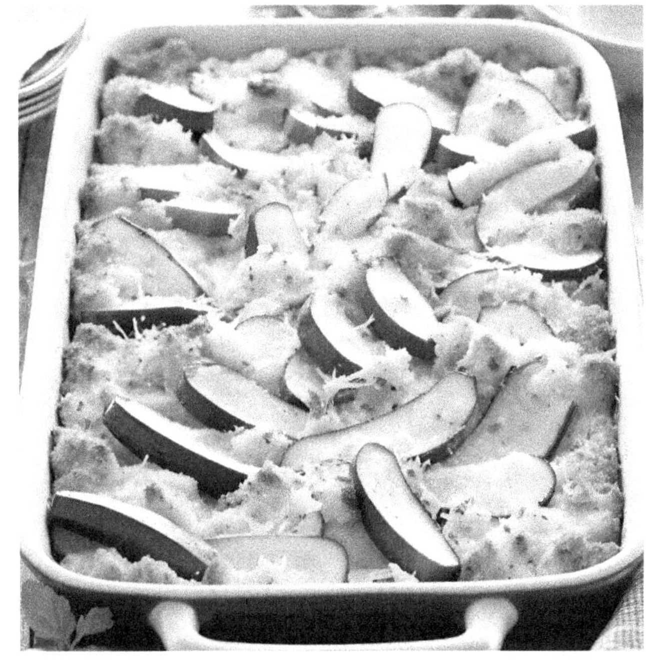

8. Greek Yogurt with Nuts and Cinnamon

Ingredients:

- 1 cup full-fat Greek yogurt
- 2 tablespoons chopped walnuts
- 2 tablespoons chopped almonds
- 1 tablespoon chia seeds
- 1 teaspoon ground cinnamon
- 1 teaspoon vanilla extract
- 1 tablespoon sugar-free sweetener (optional)

Instructions:

1. In a mixing bowl, combine the Greek yogurt, vanilla extract, and sugar-free sweetener (if using). Stir well.
2. Divide the yogurt mixture into serving bowls.
3. Top each bowl with chopped walnuts, chopped almonds, chia seeds, and ground cinnamon.
4. Serve immediately.

Nutrition Info Per Serving (1 serving):

- Calories: 280
- Total Fat: 21g
- Saturated Fat: 8g
- Cholesterol: 30mg
- Sodium: 70mg
- Total Carbohydrates: 10g
- Dietary Fiber: 5g
- Sugars: 4g
- Protein: 15g

Number of Servings: 2

Cooking Time: 5 minutes

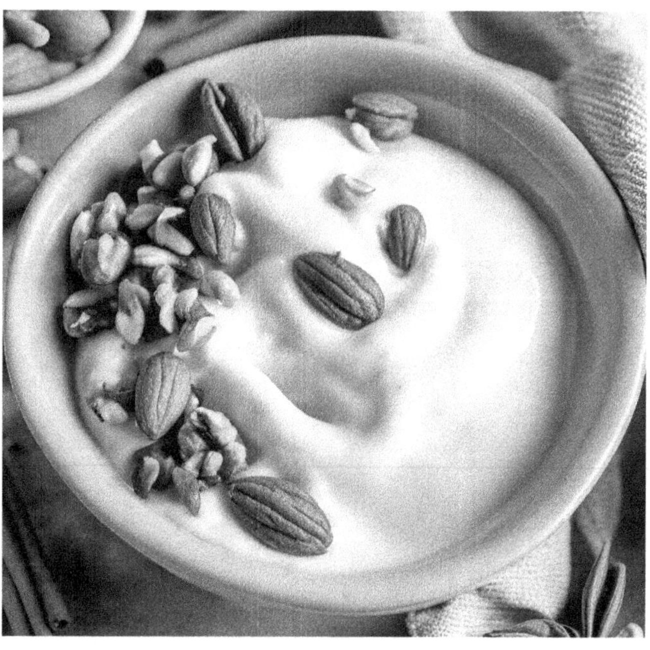

9. Almond Flour Pancakes

Ingredients:

- 1 cup almond flour
- 2 large eggs
- 1/4 cup unsweetened almond milk
- 2 tablespoons melted coconut oil
- 1 tablespoon erythritol or other sugar-free sweetener
- 1 teaspoon baking powder
- 1 teaspoon vanilla extract
- 1/2 teaspoon ground cinnamon

Instructions:

1. In a mixing bowl, whisk together the almond flour, erythritol, baking powder, and ground cinnamon.
2. In another bowl, whisk the eggs, almond milk, melted coconut oil, and vanilla extract until well combined.
3. Pour the wet ingredients into the dry ingredients and stir until smooth.
4. Heat a non-stick skillet over medium heat and lightly grease with additional coconut oil.
5. Pour 1/4 cup of batter onto the skillet for each pancake. Cook until bubbles form on the surface and the edges are set, about 2-3 minutes. Flip and cook for another 2-3 minutes, until golden brown.
6. Repeat with the remaining batter.
7. Serve warm with a topping of your choice, such as butter or a small amount of sugar-free syrup.

Nutrition Info Per Serving (2 pancakes):

- Calories: 220
- Total Fat: 18g
- Saturated Fat: 5g
- Cholesterol: 95mg
- Sodium: 150mg
- Total Carbohydrates: 5g
- Dietary Fiber: 3g
- Sugars: 1g
- Protein: 8g

Number of Servings: 4
Cooking Time: 15 minutes

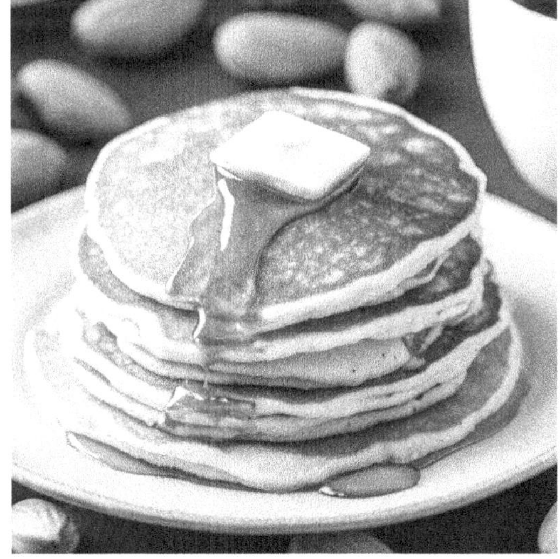

10. Avocado and Egg Breakfast Pizza

Ingredients:

- 1 large avocado, mashed
- 2 large eggs
- 1/2 cup shredded mozzarella cheese
- 1/4 cup grated Parmesan cheese
- 1/4 cup heavy cream
- 1 teaspoon garlic powder
- 1 teaspoon dried oregano
- 1 tablespoon olive oil

Instructions:

1. Preheat your oven to 375°F (190°C).
2. In a mixing bowl, combine the mashed avocado, shredded mozzarella cheese, grated Parmesan cheese, heavy cream, garlic powder, and dried oregano.
3. Grease a baking dish or a small pizza pan with olive oil.
4. Spread the avocado mixture evenly on the baking dish, forming a pizza crust.
5. Crack the eggs on top of the avocado mixture, spacing them evenly.
6. Bake in the preheated oven for 12-15 minutes, until the eggs are set to your desired doneness.
7. Remove from the oven and let cool slightly before slicing and serving.

Nutrition Info Per Serving (1 slice):

- Calories: 300
- Total Fat: 26g
- Saturated Fat: 10g
- Cholesterol: 200mg
- Sodium: 250mg
- Total Carbohydrates: 6g
- Dietary Fiber: 4g
- Sugars: 1g
- Protein: 12g

Number of Servings: 2
Cooking Time: 15 minutes

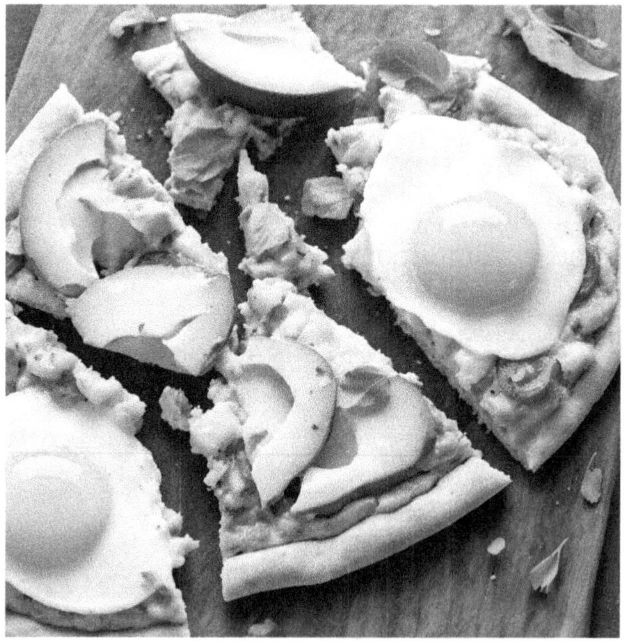

11. Beef and Egg Breakfast Muffins

Ingredients:

- 1 lb ground beef
- 6 large eggs
- 1/2 cup shredded cheddar cheese
- 1/4 cup heavy cream
- 1/4 cup chopped green onions
- 1 teaspoon garlic powder
- 1 teaspoon smoked paprika
- 1 tablespoon olive oil

Instructions:

1. Preheat your oven to 350°F (175°C).
2. Heat the olive oil in a skillet over medium-high heat. Add the ground beef and cook until browned, breaking it up into small pieces as it cooks.
3. In a mixing bowl, whisk together the eggs, heavy cream, garlic powder, and smoked paprika.
4. Grease a muffin tin with olive oil or cooking spray.
5. Divide the cooked ground beef evenly among the muffin cups.
6. Pour the egg mixture over the ground beef in each muffin cup.
7. Sprinkle the shredded cheddar cheese and chopped green onions on top.
8. Bake in the preheated oven for 15-20 minutes, or until the eggs are set and the cheese is melted and bubbly.
9. Let the muffins cool slightly before removing from the tin and serving.

Nutrition Info Per Serving (1 muffin):

- Calories: 250
- Total Fat: 20g
- Saturated Fat: 9g
- Cholesterol: 160mg
- Sodium: 220mg
- Total Carbohydrates: 2g
- Dietary Fiber: 0g
- Sugars: 0g
- Protein: 15g

Number of Servings: 6
Cooking Time: 20 minutes

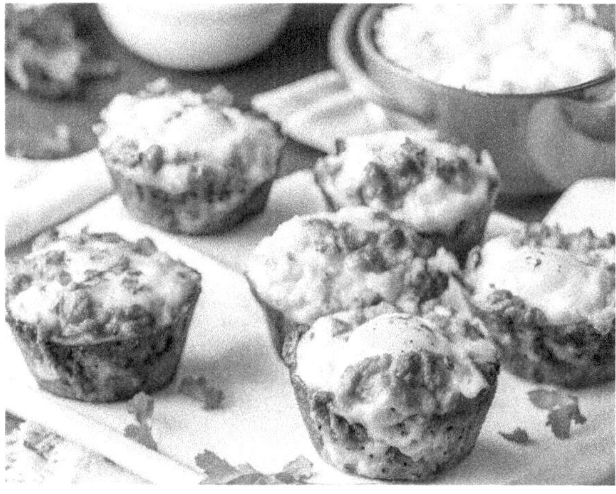

12. Keto Smoothie

Ingredients:

- 1 cup full-fat coconut milk
- 1/2 avocado
- 2 tablespoons chia seeds
- 2 tablespoons almond butter
- 1 tablespoon cocoa powder (unsweetened)
- 1 teaspoon vanilla extract
- 1 tablespoon erythritol or other sugar-free sweetener
- 1/2 cup ice cubes

Instructions:

1. Place all the ingredients in a blender: coconut milk, avocado, chia seeds, almond butter, cocoa powder, vanilla extract, erythritol, and ice cubes.
2. Blend on high until smooth and creamy.
3. Pour into a glass and serve immediately.

Nutrition Info Per Serving (1 smoothie):

- Calories: 450
- Total Fat: 38g
- Saturated Fat: 15g
- Cholesterol: 0mg
- Sodium: 60mg
- Total Carbohydrates: 14g
- Dietary Fiber: 10g
- Sugars: 1g
- Protein: 8g

Number of Servings: 1
Cooking Time: 5 minutes

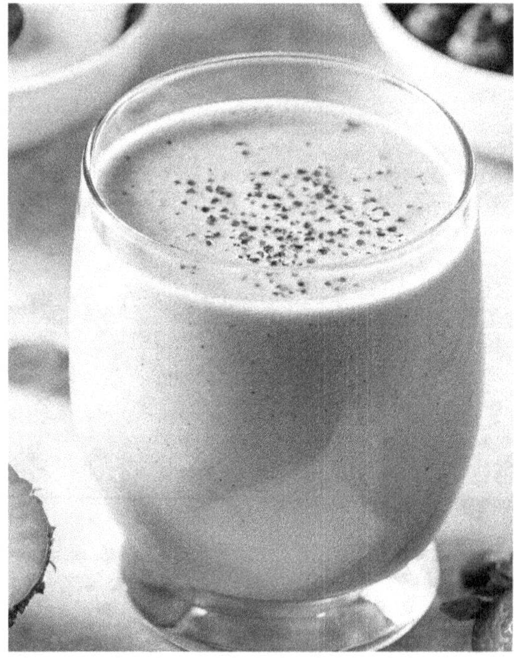

13. Ham and Cheese Stuffed Peppers

Ingredients:

- 4 large bell peppers (any color)
- 8 oz ham, diced
- 1 cup shredded cheddar cheese
- 1/2 cup cream cheese, softened
- 1/4 cup heavy cream
- 1 tablespoon Dijon mustard
- 1 tablespoon olive oil
- 1 teaspoon garlic powder
- 1 teaspoon dried oregano

Instructions:

1. Preheat your oven to 375°F (190°C).
2. Cut the tops off the bell peppers and remove the seeds and membranes.
3. In a mixing bowl, combine the diced ham, shredded cheddar cheese, cream cheese, heavy cream, Dijon mustard, garlic powder, and dried oregano. Mix until well combined.
4. Stuff each bell pepper with the ham and cheese mixture.
5. Place the stuffed peppers in a baking dish and drizzle with olive oil.
6. Bake in the preheated oven for 25-30 minutes, or until the peppers are tender and the cheese is melted and bubbly.
7. Let cool slightly before serving.

Nutrition Info Per Serving (1 stuffed pepper):

- Calories: 320
- Total Fat: 24g
- Saturated Fat: 12g
- Cholesterol: 80mg
- Sodium: 500mg
- Total Carbohydrates: 10g
- Dietary Fiber: 3g
- Sugars: 5g
- Protein: 18g

Number of Servings: 4
Cooking Time: 30 minutes

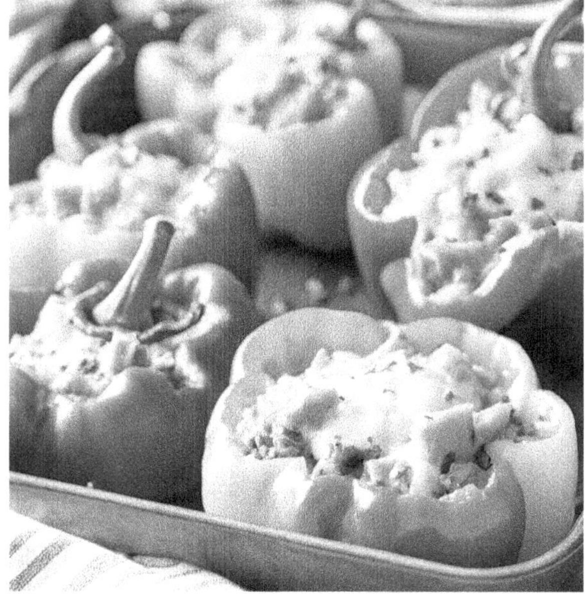

14. Coconut Flour Crepes
Ingredients:

- 4 large eggs
- 1/4 cup coconut flour
- 1/4 cup heavy cream
- 1/4 cup water
- 2 tablespoons melted butter
- 1 teaspoon vanilla extract
- 1 tablespoon erythritol or other sugar-free sweetener
- 1/2 teaspoon baking powder

Instructions:

1. In a large mixing bowl, whisk together the eggs, heavy cream, water, melted butter, vanilla extract, and erythritol until smooth.
2. Gradually add the coconut flour and baking powder, whisking until the batter is smooth and lump-free.
3. Heat a non-stick skillet over medium heat and lightly grease with additional melted butter.
4. Pour 1/4 cup of batter onto the skillet, spreading it thinly to form a crepe.
5. Cook for 2-3 minutes, until the edges start to lift and the bottom is golden brown. Flip and cook for an additional 1-2 minutes.
6. Repeat with the remaining batter.
7. Serve the crepes warm with your choice of toppings, such as whipped cream or fresh berries.

Nutrition Info Per Serving (2 crepes):

- Calories: 150
- Total Fat: 12g
- Saturated Fat: 7g
- Cholesterol: 130mg
- Sodium: 60mg
- Total Carbohydrates: 4g
- Dietary Fiber: 2g
- Sugars: 1g
- Protein: 6g

Number of Servings: 4
Cooking Time: 15 minutes

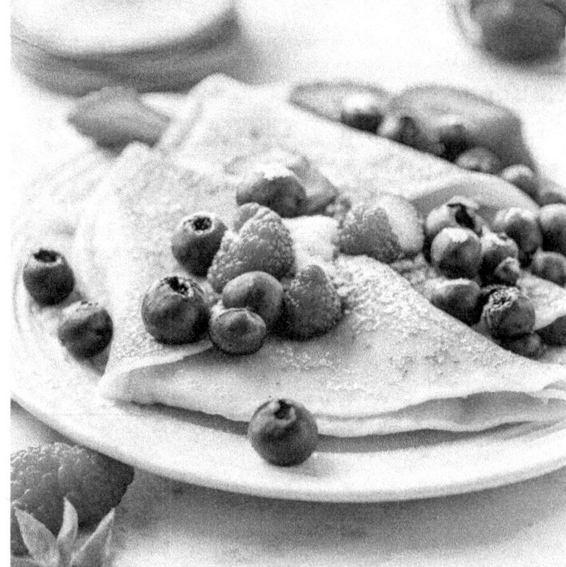

15. Pumpkin Seed Granola

Ingredients:

- 1 cup pumpkin seeds
- 1/2 cup sunflower seeds
- 1/2 cup unsweetened coconut flakes
- 1/4 cup chia seeds
- 1/4 cup flaxseeds
- 1/4 cup coconut oil, melted
- 2 tablespoons erythritol or other sugar-free sweetener
- 1 teaspoon vanilla extract
- 1 teaspoon ground cinnamon
- 1/2 teaspoon ground nutmeg

Instructions:

1. Preheat your oven to 300°F (150°C).
2. In a large mixing bowl, combine the pumpkin seeds, sunflower seeds, coconut flakes, chia seeds, and flaxseeds.
3. In a small bowl, whisk together the melted coconut oil, erythritol, vanilla extract, ground cinnamon, and ground nutmeg.
4. Pour the coconut oil mixture over the seed mixture and stir until well combined.
5. Spread the mixture evenly on a baking sheet lined with parchment paper.
6. Bake in the preheated oven for 20-25 minutes, stirring halfway through, until the granola is golden and crispy.
7. Let the granola cool completely before serving or storing in an airtight container.

Nutrition Info Per Serving (1/2 cup):

- Calories: 280
- Total Fat: 24g
- Saturated Fat: 10g
- Cholesterol: 0mg
- Sodium: 10mg
- Total Carbohydrates: 8g
- Dietary Fiber: 6g
- Sugars: 1g
- Protein: 10g

Number of Servings: 6
Cooking Time: 25 minutes

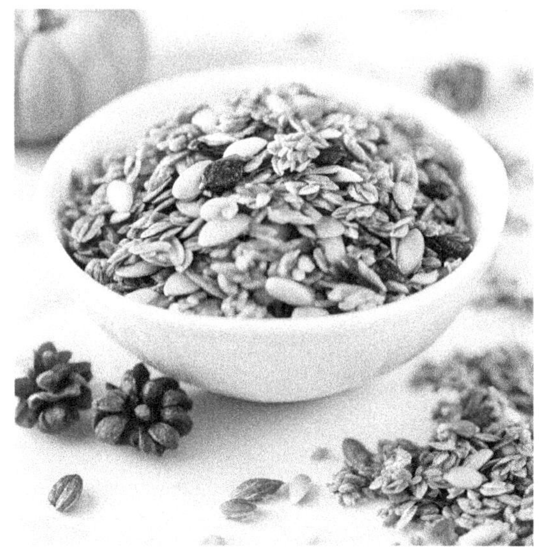

16. Cottage Cheese and Flaxseed
Ingredients:
- 1 cup full-fat cottage cheese
- 2 tablespoons ground flaxseed
- 1 tablespoon chia seeds
- 1 tablespoon chopped walnuts
- 1 teaspoon vanilla extract
- 1/2 teaspoon ground cinnamon

Instructions:
1. In a mixing bowl, combine the cottage cheese, ground flaxseed, chia seeds, chopped walnuts, vanilla extract, and ground cinnamon.
2. Stir well until all the ingredients are evenly mixed.
3. Serve immediately, or refrigerate for up to 2 hours to allow the chia seeds to soften and thicken the mixture.

Nutrition Info Per Serving (1/2 cup):
- Calories: 210
- Total Fat: 14g
- Saturated Fat: 6g
- Cholesterol: 30mg
- Sodium: 350mg
- Total Carbohydrates: 7g
- Dietary Fiber: 4g
- Sugars: 2g
- Protein: 14g

Number of Servings: 2 Cooking Time: 5 minutes

17. Eggplant and Feta Bake

Ingredients:

- 1 large eggplant, sliced into rounds
- 1/2 cup crumbled feta cheese
- 1/2 cup shredded mozzarella cheese
- 1/4 cup olive oil
- 1/4 cup heavy cream
- 2 cloves garlic, minced
- 1 teaspoon dried oregano
- 1 teaspoon dried thyme

Instructions:

1. Preheat your oven to 375°F (190°C).
2. Lightly grease a baking dish with olive oil.
3. Arrange the eggplant slices in a single layer in the baking dish.
4. In a small bowl, mix the olive oil, heavy cream, minced garlic, oregano, and thyme.
5. Drizzle the olive oil mixture over the eggplant slices.
6. Sprinkle the crumbled feta cheese and shredded mozzarella cheese evenly over the eggplant.
7. Bake in the preheated oven for 25-30 minutes, until the eggplant is tender and the cheese is melted and golden.
8. Let cool slightly before serving.

Nutrition Info Per Serving (1 serving):

- Calories: 220
- Total Fat: 19g
- Saturated Fat: 8g
- Cholesterol: 35mg
- Sodium: 320mg
- Total Carbohydrates: 6g
- Dietary Fiber: 2g
- Sugars: 3g
- Protein: 6g

Number of Servings: 4

Cooking Time: 30 minutes

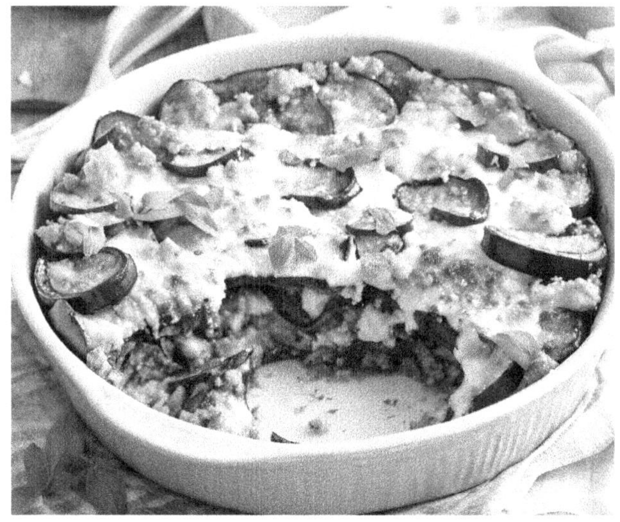

18. Keto Bagels

Ingredients:

- 2 cups almond flour
- 1 tablespoon baking powder
- 2 cups shredded mozzarella cheese
- 2 oz cream cheese
- 2 large eggs
- 1 tablespoon sesame seeds (optional)

Instructions:

1. Preheat your oven to 400°F (200°C). Line a baking sheet with parchment paper.
2. In a mixing bowl, combine the almond flour and baking powder.
3. In a microwave-safe bowl, combine the shredded mozzarella cheese and cream cheese. Microwave on high for 1-2 minutes, stirring halfway through, until the cheese is completely melted and smooth.
4. Add the melted cheese mixture to the almond flour mixture, along with the eggs. Mix until a dough forms.
5. Divide the dough into 6 equal parts and roll each part into a log shape. Form each log into a bagel shape and place on the prepared baking sheet.
6. Sprinkle the sesame seeds on top of the bagels, if using.
7. Bake in the preheated oven for 12-15 minutes, or until the bagels are golden brown.
8. Let cool before serving.

Nutrition Info Per Serving (1 bagel):

- Calories: 350
- Total Fat: 28g
- Saturated Fat: 10g
- Cholesterol: 95mg
- Sodium: 360mg
- Total Carbohydrates: 8g
- Dietary Fiber: 4g
- Sugars: 1g
- Protein: 17g

Number of Servings: 6

Cooking Time: 15 minutes

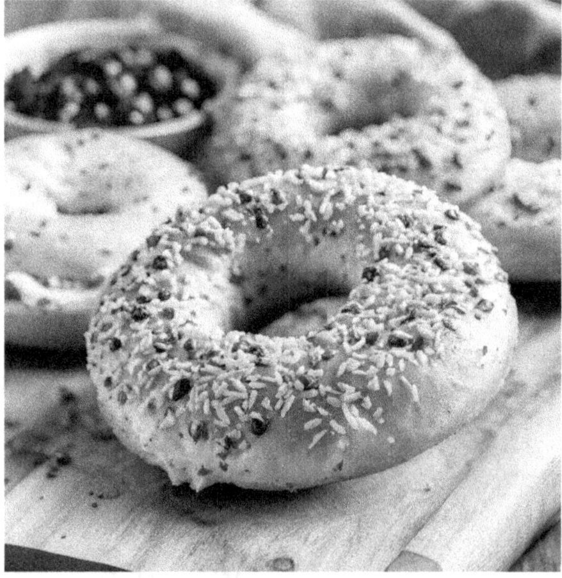

19. Cauliflower and Cheese Breakfast Porridge

Ingredients:

- 2 cups cauliflower rice
- 1 cup heavy cream
- 1/2 cup shredded cheddar cheese
- 2 tablespoons butter
- 1 teaspoon garlic powder
- 1/2 teaspoon ground nutmeg

Instructions:

1. In a medium saucepan, combine the cauliflower rice, heavy cream, garlic powder, and ground nutmeg.
2. Cook over medium heat, stirring occasionally, until the mixture begins to simmer and thicken, about 10 minutes.
3. Stir in the shredded cheddar cheese and butter. Continue to cook until the cheese is melted and the porridge reaches your desired consistency, about 5 more minutes.
4. Remove from heat and serve hot.

Nutrition Info Per Serving (1 serving):

- Calories: 320
- Total Fat: 30g
- Saturated Fat: 18g
- Cholesterol: 100mg
- Sodium: 250mg
- Total Carbohydrates: 6g
- Dietary Fiber: 2g
- Sugars: 2g
- Protein: 8g

Number of Servings: 2
Cooking Time: 15 minutes

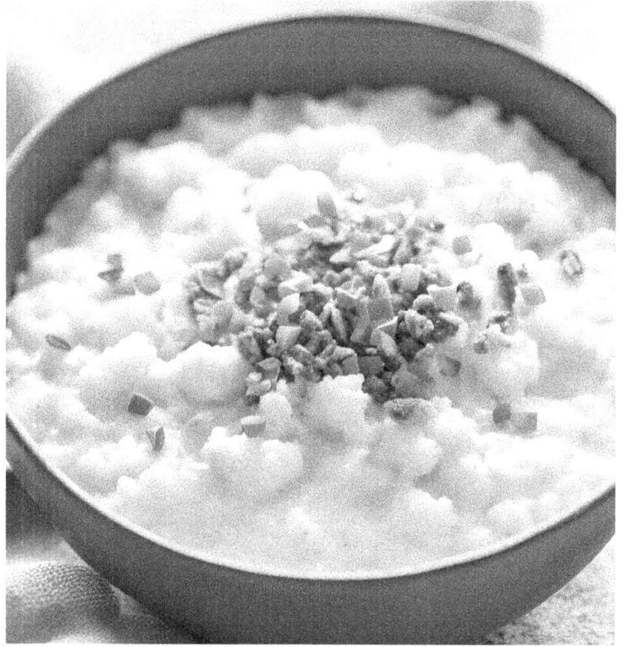

20. Bacon and Kale Stir-Fry

Ingredients:

- 6 slices bacon, chopped
- 4 cups chopped kale
- 1/2 cup sliced almonds
- 2 tablespoons olive oil
- 2 cloves garlic, minced
- 1 teaspoon dried thyme

Instructions:

1. Heat a large skillet over medium heat. Add the chopped bacon and cook until crispy, about 5-7 minutes. Remove the bacon from the skillet and set aside.
2. In the same skillet, add the olive oil and garlic. Sauté for 1 minute until fragrant.
3. Add the chopped kale and dried thyme to the skillet. Cook, stirring occasionally, until the kale is wilted and tender, about 5 minutes.
4. Stir in the cooked bacon and sliced almonds. Cook for an additional 2 minutes until everything is heated through.
5. Serve immediately.

Nutrition Info Per Serving (1 serving):

- Calories: 280
- Total Fat: 24g
- Saturated Fat: 6g
- Cholesterol: 25mg
- Sodium: 400mg
- Total Carbohydrates: 6g
- Dietary Fiber: 3g
- Sugars: 1g
- Protein: 10g

Number of Servings: 2
Cooking Time: 15 minutes

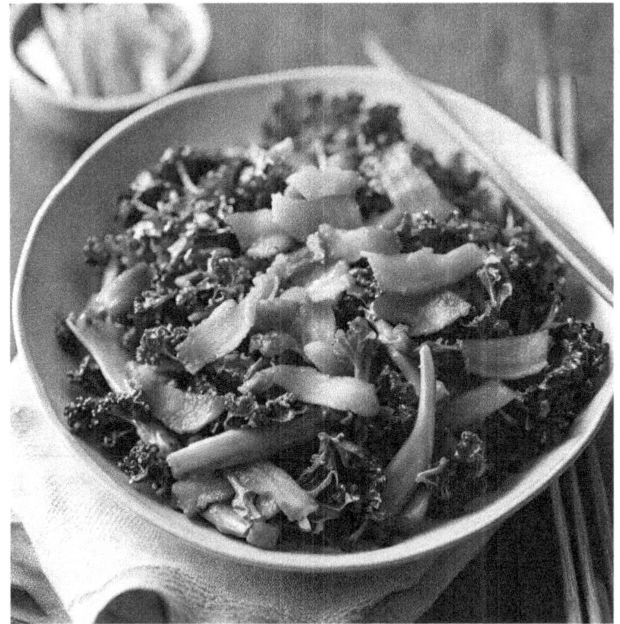

21. Mushroom and Goat Cheese Scramble

Ingredients:

- 4 large eggs
- 1/4 cup heavy cream
- 1/2 cup sliced mushrooms
- 1/4 cup crumbled goat cheese
- 2 tablespoons butter
- 1 teaspoon dried basil
- 1 teaspoon garlic powder

Instructions:

1. In a mixing bowl, whisk together the eggs, heavy cream, dried basil, and garlic powder.
2. Heat the butter in a non-stick skillet over medium heat. Add the sliced mushrooms and sauté until tender, about 5 minutes.
3. Pour the egg mixture into the skillet with the mushrooms. Cook, stirring occasionally, until the eggs are scrambled and just set, about 3-4 minutes.
4. Remove from heat and gently fold in the crumbled goat cheese.
5. Serve immediately.

Nutrition Info Per Serving (1 serving):

- Calories: 300
- Total Fat: 26g
- Saturated Fat: 13g
- Cholesterol: 260mg
- Sodium: 200mg
- Total Carbohydrates: 3g
- Dietary Fiber: 1g
- Sugars: 1g
- Protein: 13g

Number of Servings: 2
Cooking Time: 10 minutes

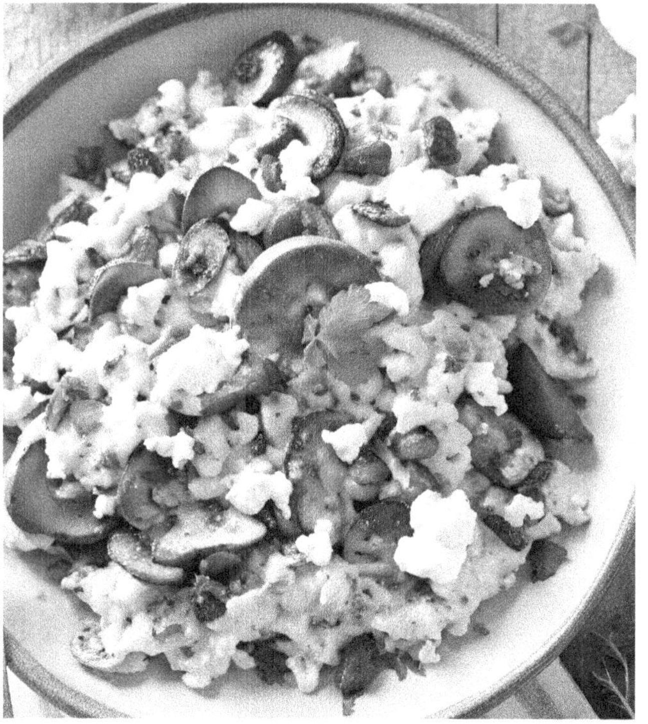

22. Broccoli and Cheddar Quiche

Ingredients:

- 1 cup chopped broccoli florets
- 1 cup shredded cheddar cheese
- 6 large eggs
- 1/2 cup heavy cream
- 1/4 cup grated Parmesan cheese
- 2 tablespoons butter
- 1 teaspoon garlic powder
- 1 teaspoon dried thyme

Instructions:

1. Preheat your oven to 375°F (190°C).
2. In a large skillet, melt the butter over medium heat. Add the chopped broccoli and cook until tender, about 5 minutes. Set aside to cool slightly.
3. In a mixing bowl, whisk together the eggs, heavy cream, garlic powder, and dried thyme.
4. Add the cooked broccoli, shredded cheddar cheese, and grated Parmesan cheese to the egg mixture. Stir to combine.
5. Pour the mixture into a greased 9-inch pie dish.
6. Bake in the preheated oven for 25-30 minutes, or until the quiche is set and the top is golden brown.
7. Let cool slightly before slicing and serving.

Nutrition Info Per Serving (1 slice):

- Calories: 320
- Total Fat: 27g
- Saturated Fat: 15g
- Cholesterol: 225mg
- Sodium: 320mg
- Total Carbohydrates: 4g
- Dietary Fiber: 1g
- Sugars: 1g
- Protein: 15g

Number of Servings: 6

Cooking Time: 30 minutes

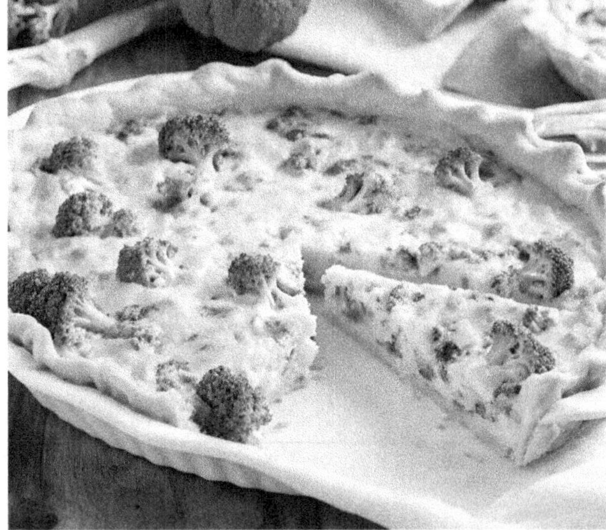

23. Ricotta and Walnut Cream

Ingredients:

- 1 cup full-fat ricotta cheese
- 1/4 cup heavy cream
- 1/4 cup finely chopped walnuts
- 1 tablespoon erythritol or other sugar-free sweetener
- 1 teaspoon vanilla extract
- 1/2 teaspoon ground cinnamon

Instructions:

1. In a mixing bowl, combine the ricotta cheese, heavy cream, erythritol, vanilla extract, and ground cinnamon. Mix until smooth and creamy.
2. Gently fold in the finely chopped walnuts.
3. Serve immediately, or refrigerate for up to 2 hours before serving.

Nutrition Info Per Serving (1/2 cup):

- Calories: 300
- Total Fat: 25g
- Saturated Fat: 13g
- Cholesterol: 70mg
- Sodium: 80mg
- Total Carbohydrates: 5g
- Dietary Fiber: 1g
- Sugars: 2g
- Protein: 10g

Number of Servings: 2 Cooking Time: 5 minutes

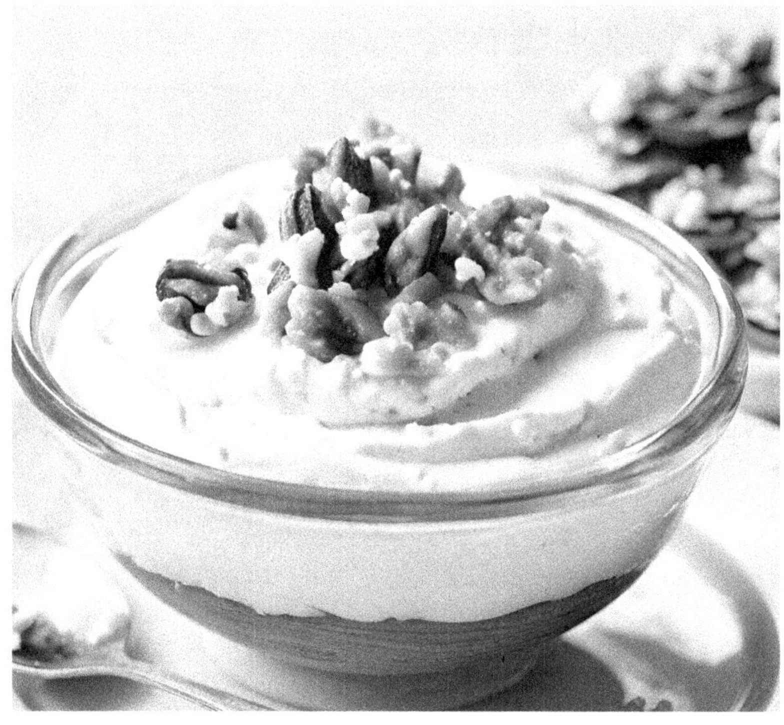

24. Lemon and Poppy Seed Muffins

Ingredients:

- 2 cups almond flour
- 1/4 cup coconut flour
- 1/2 cup erythritol or other sugar-free sweetener
- 1/4 cup poppy seeds
- 1/2 cup melted coconut oil
- 4 large eggs
- 1/2 cup heavy cream
- 2 tablespoons lemon zest
- 2 tablespoons lemon juice
- 1 teaspoon baking powder
- 1 teaspoon vanilla extract

Instructions:

1. Preheat your oven to 350°F (175°C). Line a muffin tin with paper liners.
2. In a large mixing bowl, whisk together the almond flour, coconut flour, erythritol, poppy seeds, and baking powder.
3. In another bowl, whisk the eggs, melted coconut oil, heavy cream, lemon zest, lemon juice, and vanilla extract until well combined.
4. Pour the wet ingredients into the dry ingredients and stir until just combined.
5. Divide the batter evenly among the muffin cups.
6. Bake in the preheated oven for 20-25 minutes, or until a toothpick inserted into the center comes out clean.
7. Let the muffins cool in the tin for 5 minutes before transferring to a wire rack to cool completely.

Nutrition Info Per Serving (1 muffin):

- Calories: 210
- Total Fat: 18g
- Saturated Fat: 8g
- Cholesterol: 70mg
- Sodium: 80mg
- Total Carbohydrates: 6g
- Dietary Fiber: 3g
- Sugars: 1g
- Protein: 6g

Number of Servings: 12
Cooking Time: 25 minutes

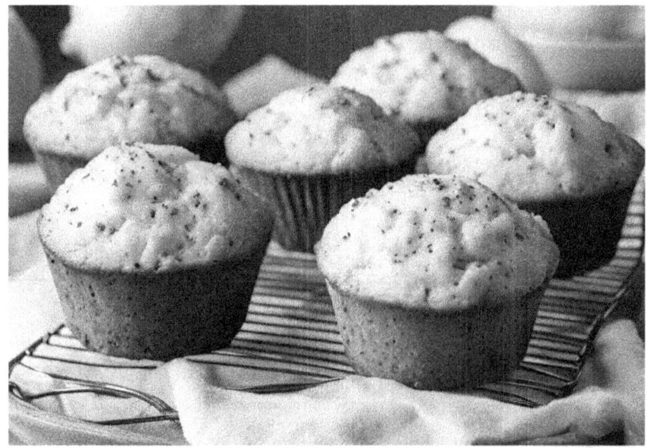

25. Butter-Fried Green Cabbage

Ingredients:

- 4 cups shredded green cabbage
- 4 tablespoons butter
- 1/2 cup heavy cream
- 1 teaspoon garlic powder
- 1 teaspoon dried thyme

Instructions:

1. In a large skillet, melt the butter over medium-high heat.
2. Add the shredded cabbage to the skillet and cook, stirring occasionally, until the cabbage is tender and slightly caramelized, about 10-15 minutes.
3. Reduce the heat to medium and stir in the heavy cream, garlic powder, and dried thyme.
4. Cook for an additional 3-5 minutes, until the cream has thickened and the cabbage is well-coated.
5. Serve hot.

Nutrition Info Per Serving (1 cup):

- Calories: 250
- Total Fat: 22g
- Saturated Fat: 14g
- Cholesterol: 70mg
- Sodium: 80mg
- Total Carbohydrates: 8g
- Dietary Fiber: 4g
- Sugars: 4g
- Protein: 3g

Number of Servings: 4
Cooking Time: 20 minutes

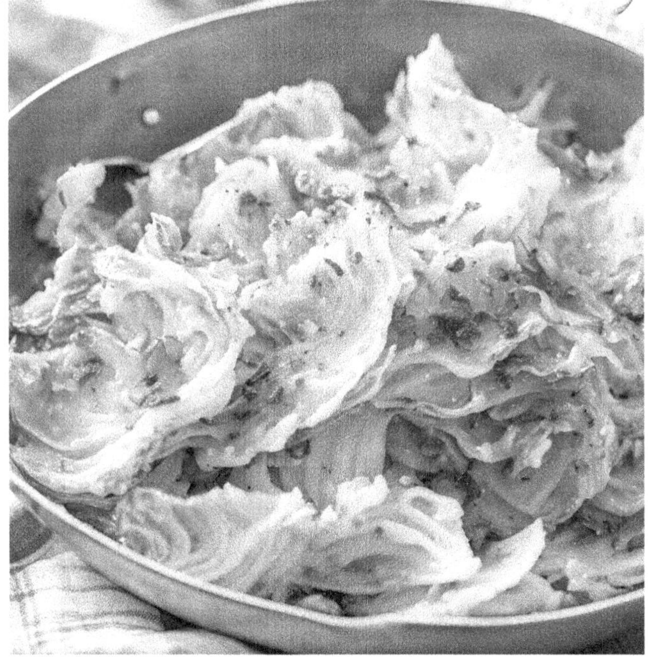

25. Egg and Olive Tapenade Tartines

Ingredients:

- 4 large hard-boiled eggs
- 1/2 cup black olive tapenade
- 4 slices of low-carb bread
- 2 tablespoons mayonnaise (preferably made with avocado oil)
- 1 tablespoon olive oil
- 1 teaspoon dried oregano
- 1 tablespoon chopped fresh parsley

Instructions:

1. Peel and slice the hard-boiled eggs.
2. Toast the low-carb bread slices to your desired level of crispiness.
3. Spread a thin layer of mayonnaise on each slice of toasted bread.
4. Arrange the egg slices evenly on top of the mayonnaise.
5. Spread the olive tapenade over the eggs.
6. Drizzle with olive oil and sprinkle with dried oregano.
7. Garnish with chopped fresh parsley.
8. Serve immediately.

Nutrition Info Per Serving (1 tartine):

- Calories: 280
- Total Fat: 24g
- Saturated Fat: 5g
- Cholesterol: 210mg
- Sodium: 450mg
- Total Carbohydrates: 4g
- Dietary Fiber: 1g
- Sugars: 1g
- Protein: 10g

Number of Servings: 4
Cooking Time: 10 minutes

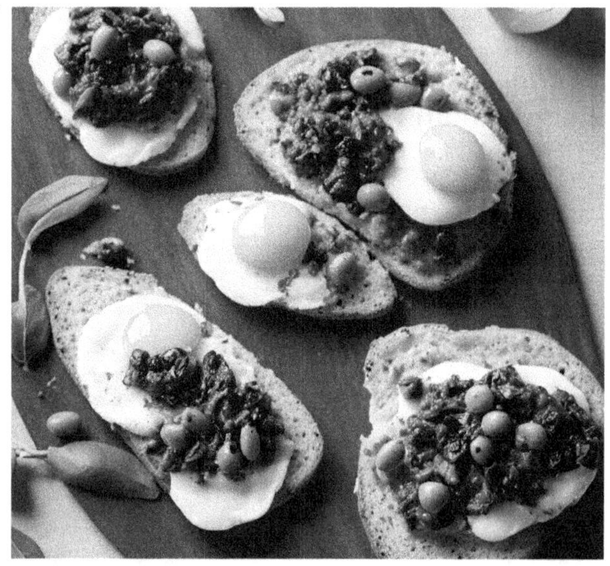

26. Cinnamon Bun Smoothie

Ingredients:

- 1 cup unsweetened almond milk
- 1/2 avocado
- 2 tablespoons chia seeds
- 1 tablespoon almond butter
- 1 tablespoon erythritol or other sugar-free sweetener
- 1 teaspoon vanilla extract
- 1 teaspoon ground cinnamon
- 1/4 teaspoon ground nutmeg
- 1/4 teaspoon ground cloves
- 1/2 cup ice cubes

Instructions:

1. Place all the ingredients in a blender: almond milk, avocado, chia seeds, almond butter, erythritol, vanilla extract, ground cinnamon, ground nutmeg, ground cloves, and ice cubes.
2. Blend on high until smooth and creamy.
3. Pour into a glass and serve immediately.

Nutrition Info Per Serving (1 smoothie):

- Calories: 320
- Total Fat: 28g
- Saturated Fat: 3g
- Cholesterol: 0mg
- Sodium: 70mg
- Total Carbohydrates: 12g
- Dietary Fiber: 8g
- Sugars: 1g
- Protein: 7g

Number of Servings: 1
Cooking Time: 5 minutes

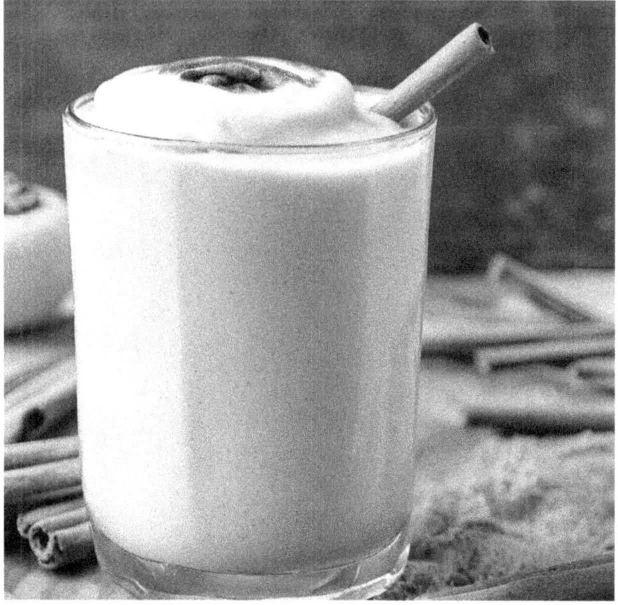

27. Cheese and Walnut Balls

Ingredients:

- 1 cup cream cheese, softened
- 1 cup shredded sharp cheddar cheese
- 1/2 cup finely chopped walnuts
- 1 tablespoon chopped fresh chives
- 1 teaspoon garlic powder
- 1 teaspoon dried dill

Instructions:

1. In a mixing bowl, combine the cream cheese, shredded cheddar cheese, chopped walnuts, chopped fresh chives, garlic powder, and dried dill. Mix until well combined.
2. Form the mixture into small balls, about 1 inch in diameter.
3. Place the cheese balls on a plate and refrigerate for at least 1 hour to firm up.
4. Serve chilled.

Nutrition Info Per Serving (2 cheese balls):

- Calories: 200
- Total Fat: 18g
- Saturated Fat: 8g
- Cholesterol: 40mg
- Sodium: 180mg
- Total Carbohydrates: 2g
- Dietary Fiber: 1g
- Sugars: 0g
- Protein: 6g

Number of Servings: 8

Cooking Time: 10 minutes (plus 1 hour chilling time)

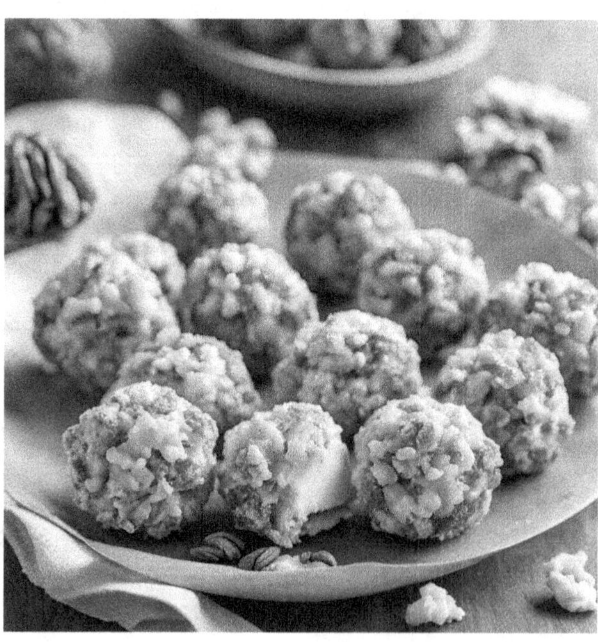

Beef and Pork Recipes

1. Beef Steak with Herb Butter

Ingredients:

- 4 beef ribeye steaks (8 oz each)
- 1/2 cup unsalted butter, softened
- 2 tablespoons chopped fresh parsley
- 1 tablespoon chopped fresh rosemary
- 1 tablespoon chopped fresh thyme
- 2 cloves garlic, minced
- 2 tablespoons olive oil

Instructions:

1. In a small bowl, combine the softened butter, chopped parsley, rosemary, thyme, and minced garlic. Mix well to create the herb butter. Set aside.
2. Heat a large skillet or grill pan over medium-high heat. Add the olive oil and allow it to heat up.
3. Add the ribeye steaks to the skillet and cook for 4-5 minutes on each side for medium-rare, or until they reach your desired level of doneness.
4. Remove the steaks from the skillet and let them rest for 5 minutes.
5. Top each steak with a generous dollop of herb butter.
6. Serve immediately.

Nutrition Info Per Serving (1 steak with herb butter):

- Calories: 600
- Total Fat: 52g
- Saturated Fat: 24g
- Cholesterol: 160mg
- Sodium: 120mg
- Total Carbohydrates: 1g
- Dietary Fiber: 0g
- Sugars: 0g
- Protein: 34g

Number of Servings: 4
Cooking Time: 15 minutes

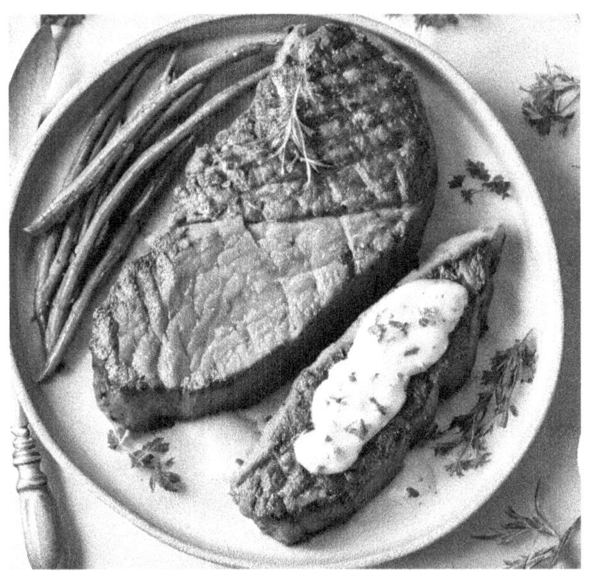

2. Pork Chops with Creamy Mushroom Sauce

Ingredients:

- 4 bone-in pork chops (8 oz each)
- 2 tablespoons olive oil
- 1 cup heavy cream
- 1 cup sliced mushrooms
- 1/2 cup grated Parmesan cheese
- 2 cloves garlic, minced
- 1 teaspoon dried thyme

Instructions:

1. Heat the olive oil in a large skillet over medium-high heat.
2. Add the pork chops to the skillet and cook for 4-5 minutes on each side, until golden brown and cooked through. Remove the pork chops from the skillet and set aside.
3. In the same skillet, add the minced garlic and sliced mushrooms. Sauté for 2-3 minutes until the mushrooms are tender.
4. Reduce the heat to medium and add the heavy cream, grated Parmesan cheese, and dried thyme to the skillet. Stir well to combine.
5. Simmer the sauce for 3-4 minutes, until it thickens.
6. Return the pork chops to the skillet and spoon the creamy mushroom sauce over them.
7. Serve immediately.

Nutrition Info Per Serving (1 pork chop with sauce):

- Calories: 550
- Total Fat: 44g
- Saturated Fat: 20g
- Cholesterol: 150mg
- Sodium: 220mg
- Total Carbohydrates: 4g
- Dietary Fiber: 1g
- Sugars: 1g
- Protein: 36g

Number of Servings: 4

Cooking Time: 20 minutes

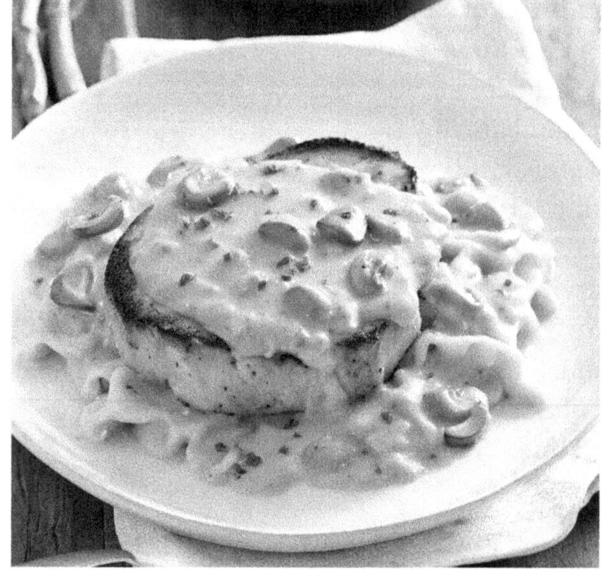

3. Slow Cooker Beef Brisket

Ingredients:

- 4 lbs beef brisket
- 1/4 cup olive oil
- 1 cup beef broth
- 1/2 cup Worcestershire sauce
- 1/4 cup apple cider vinegar
- 4 cloves garlic, minced
- 1 tablespoon smoked paprika
- 1 tablespoon onion powder
- 1 teaspoon dried oregano
- 1 teaspoon dried thyme

Instructions:

1. In a small bowl, mix the smoked paprika, onion powder, dried oregano, and dried thyme.
2. Rub the spice mixture all over the beef brisket.
3. Heat the olive oil in a large skillet over medium-high heat. Sear the brisket on all sides until browned, about 4-5 minutes per side.
4. Transfer the seared brisket to a slow cooker.
5. In the same skillet, add the minced garlic and sauté for 1 minute until fragrant.
6. Add the beef broth, Worcestershire sauce, and apple cider vinegar to the skillet. Stir well and bring to a simmer.
7. Pour the sauce over the brisket in the slow cooker.
8. Cover and cook on low for 8-10 hours, until the brisket is tender.
9. Remove the brisket from the slow cooker and let it rest for 10 minutes before slicing.
10. Serve with the cooking juices spooned over the top.

Nutrition Info Per Serving (1 serving of brisket):

- Calories: 500
- Total Fat: 36g
- Saturated Fat: 12g
- Cholesterol: 140mg
- Sodium: 380mg
- Total Carbohydrates: 3g
- Dietary Fiber: 0g
- Sugars: 1g
- Protein: 38g

Number of Servings: 8

Cooking Time: 10 hours (slow cooker)

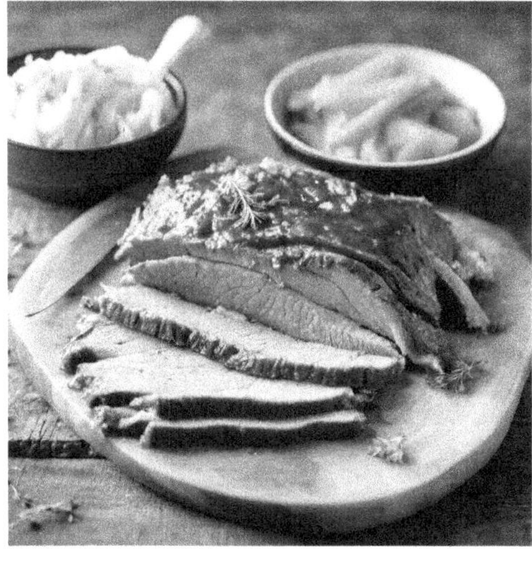

4. Beef Ribs with Spicy Rub

Ingredients:

- 4 lbs beef ribs
- 2 tablespoons olive oil
- 2 tablespoons smoked paprika
- 1 tablespoon garlic powder
- 1 tablespoon onion powder
- 1 tablespoon ground cumin
- 1 teaspoon ground cayenne pepper
- 1 teaspoon dried oregano
- 1 teaspoon dried thyme

Instructions:

1. Preheat your oven to 300°F (150°C).
2. In a small bowl, mix together the smoked paprika, garlic powder, onion powder, ground cumin, ground cayenne pepper, dried oregano, and dried thyme.
3. Rub the spice mixture evenly over the beef ribs.
4. Drizzle the olive oil over the ribs and rub it in to help the spices adhere.
5. Place the ribs on a baking sheet lined with foil.
6. Cover the ribs with another piece of foil and seal the edges.
7. Bake in the preheated oven for 3-3.5 hours, until the ribs are tender.
8. Remove the top piece of foil and increase the oven temperature to 400°F (200°C).
9. Bake for an additional 10-15 minutes to crisp up the surface.
10. Let the ribs rest for a few minutes before serving.

Nutrition Info Per Serving (1 serving):

- Calories: 520
- Total Fat: 42g
- Saturated Fat: 16g
- Cholesterol: 140mg
- Sodium: 120mg
- Total Carbohydrates: 3g
- Dietary Fiber: 1g
- Sugars: 1g
- Protein: 30g

Number of Servings: 6

Cooking Time: 3.5-4 hours

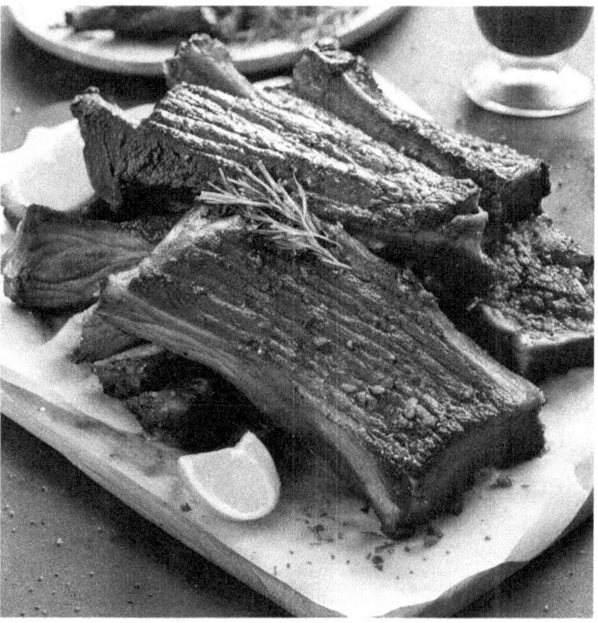

5. Pork Belly with Crispy Skin

Ingredients:

- 2 lbs pork belly, skin on
- 1 tablespoon olive oil
- 1 teaspoon garlic powder
- 1 teaspoon onion powder
- 1 teaspoon smoked paprika
- 1 teaspoon dried rosemary

Instructions:

1. Preheat your oven to 350°F (175°C).
2. Score the skin of the pork belly in a crosshatch pattern.
3. In a small bowl, mix together the garlic powder, onion powder, smoked paprika, and dried rosemary.
4. Rub the spice mixture all over the pork belly.
5. Drizzle the olive oil over the pork belly and rub it in.
6. Place the pork belly on a rack in a roasting pan, skin-side up.
7. Roast in the preheated oven for 2 hours.
8. Increase the oven temperature to 425°F (220°C) and roast for an additional 20-30 minutes, until the skin is crispy.
9. Let the pork belly rest for 10 minutes before slicing and serving.

Nutrition Info Per Serving (1 serving):

- Calories: 600
- Total Fat: 55g
- Saturated Fat: 22g
- Cholesterol: 70mg
- Sodium: 150mg
- Total Carbohydrates: 1g
- Dietary Fiber: 0g
- Sugars: 0g
- Protein: 15g

Number of Servings: 6
Cooking Time: 2.5 hours

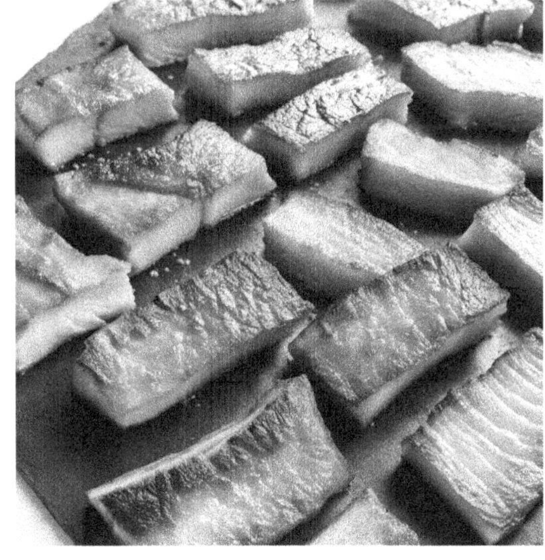

6. Keto Beef Stroganoff

Ingredients:

- 2 lbs beef sirloin, thinly sliced
- 1 cup heavy cream
- 1 cup beef broth
- 1/2 cup sour cream
- 1 cup sliced mushrooms
- 1 small onion, finely chopped
- 2 cloves garlic, minced
- 2 tablespoons olive oil
- 1 tablespoon Dijon mustard
- 1 teaspoon paprika

Instructions:

1. Heat the olive oil in a large skillet over medium-high heat.
2. Add the sliced beef and cook until browned, about 5-7 minutes. Remove the beef from the skillet and set aside.
3. In the same skillet, add the chopped onion and cook until translucent, about 3 minutes.
4. Add the minced garlic and sliced mushrooms, and cook until the mushrooms are tender, about 5 minutes.
5. Stir in the beef broth, heavy cream, Dijon mustard, and paprika. Bring to a simmer.
6. Return the beef to the skillet and simmer for 10 minutes, allowing the flavors to meld.
7. Stir in the sour cream and cook for an additional 2-3 minutes until heated through.
8. Serve immediately.

Nutrition Info Per Serving (1 serving):

- Calories: 520
- Total Fat: 42g
- Saturated Fat: 20g
- Cholesterol: 150mg
- Sodium: 280mg
- Total Carbohydrates: 5g
- Dietary Fiber: 1g
- Sugars: 2g
- Protein: 30g

Number of Servings: 6

Cooking Time: 30 minutes

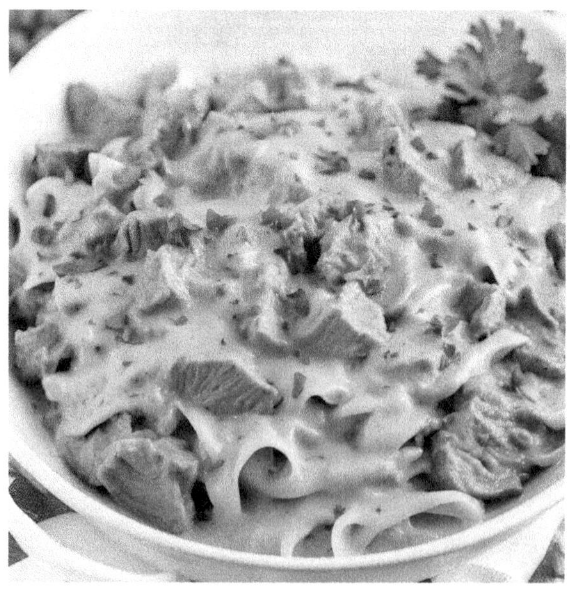

7. Stuffed Pork Tenderloin

Ingredients:

- 2 lbs pork tenderloin
- 1 cup spinach, chopped
- 1/2 cup crumbled feta cheese
- 1/4 cup sun-dried tomatoes, chopped
- 2 tablespoons olive oil
- 2 cloves garlic, minced
- 1 teaspoon dried oregano

Instructions:

1. Preheat your oven to 375°F (190°C).
2. Butterfly the pork tenderloin by cutting it lengthwise down the middle, being careful not to cut all the way through.
3. In a mixing bowl, combine the chopped spinach, crumbled feta cheese, chopped sun-dried tomatoes, minced garlic, and dried oregano.
4. Spread the spinach mixture evenly over the opened pork tenderloin.
5. Roll up the tenderloin and secure it with kitchen twine.
6. Heat the olive oil in an oven-safe skillet over medium-high heat. Sear the pork tenderloin on all sides until browned, about 5-7 minutes.
7. Transfer the skillet to the preheated oven and bake for 25-30 minutes, until the pork is cooked through.
8. Let the tenderloin rest for 10 minutes before slicing and serving.

Nutrition Info Per Serving (1 serving):

- Calories: 350
- Total Fat: 24g
- Saturated Fat: 8g
- Cholesterol: 100mg
- Sodium: 320mg
- Total Carbohydrates: 4g
- Dietary Fiber: 1g
- Sugars: 1g
- Protein: 30g

Number of Servings: 6
Cooking Time: 40 minutes

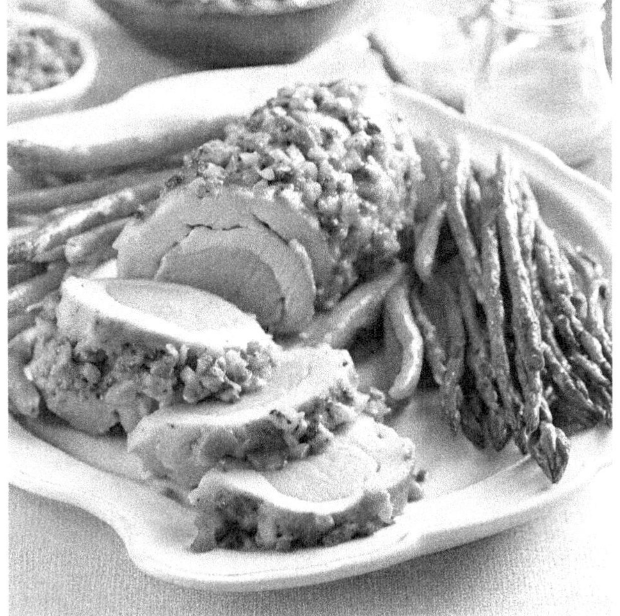

8. Spicy Pork Rinds

Ingredients:

- 4 cups pork rinds
- 2 tablespoons olive oil
- 1 teaspoon smoked paprika
- 1/2 teaspoon cayenne pepper
- 1 teaspoon garlic powder
- 1 teaspoon onion powder
- 1/2 teaspoon dried oregano

Instructions:

1. Preheat your oven to 350°F (175°C).
2. In a large mixing bowl, combine the olive oil, smoked paprika, cayenne pepper, garlic powder, onion powder, and dried oregano. Mix well.
3. Add the pork rinds to the bowl and toss until they are evenly coated with the spice mixture.
4. Spread the seasoned pork rinds in a single layer on a baking sheet.
5. Bake in the preheated oven for 5-7 minutes, until the pork rinds are crispy and the spices are fragrant.
6. Allow the pork rinds to cool slightly before serving.

Nutrition Info Per Serving (1 cup):

- Calories: 150
- Total Fat: 12g
- Saturated Fat: 2g
- Cholesterol: 20mg
- Sodium: 200mg
- Total Carbohydrates: 1g
- Dietary Fiber: 0g
- Sugars: 0g
- Protein: 9g

Number of Servings: 4
Cooking Time: 10 minutes

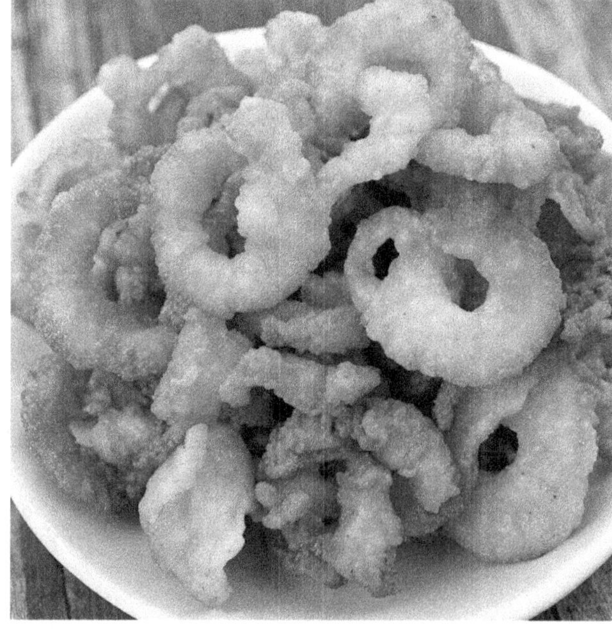

9. Bacon-Wrapped Pork Medallions

Ingredients:

- 2 lbs pork tenderloin, cut into 1-inch medallions
- 12 slices of bacon
- 2 tablespoons olive oil
- 1 tablespoon dried rosemary
- 1 tablespoon garlic powder
- 1 teaspoon ground paprika

Instructions:

1. Preheat your oven to 375°F (190°C).
2. In a small bowl, mix together the dried rosemary, garlic powder, and ground paprika.
3. Rub the spice mixture evenly over the pork medallions.
4. Wrap each pork medallion with a slice of bacon and secure with a toothpick.
5. Heat the olive oil in a large skillet over medium-high heat. Sear the bacon-wrapped medallions on both sides until browned, about 2-3 minutes per side.
6. Transfer the seared medallions to a baking sheet and bake in the preheated oven for 15-20 minutes, until the pork is cooked through and the bacon is crispy.
7. Remove the toothpicks before serving.

Nutrition Info Per Serving (2 medallions):

- Calories: 350
- Total Fat: 28g
- Saturated Fat: 10g
- Cholesterol: 90mg
- Sodium: 400mg
- Total Carbohydrates: 1g
- Dietary Fiber: 0g
- Sugars: 0g
- Protein: 22g

Number of Servings: 6
Cooking Time: 25 minutes

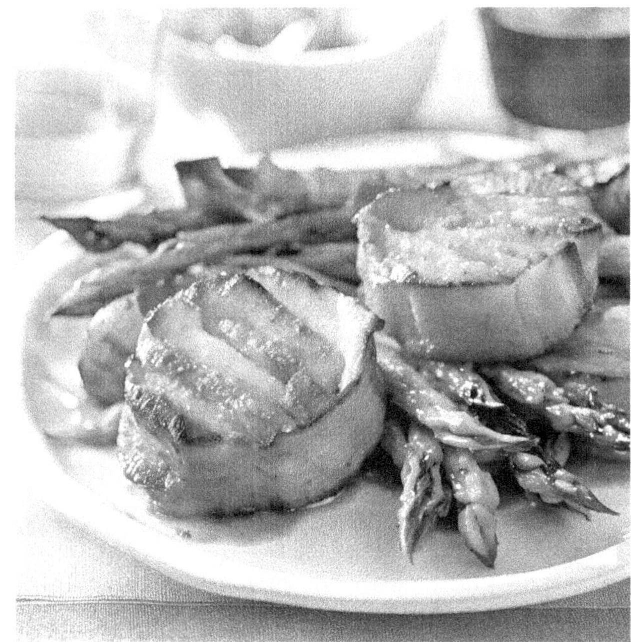

10. Italian Meatballs
Ingredients:
- 1 lb ground beef
- 1/2 lb ground pork
- 1/2 cup grated Parmesan cheese
- 1/4 cup almond flour
- 1/4 cup heavy cream
- 1 large egg
- 2 cloves garlic, minced
- 1 tablespoon dried oregano
- 1 tablespoon dried basil
- 1 teaspoon ground paprika

Instructions:
1. Preheat your oven to 375°F (190°C).
2. In a large mixing bowl, combine the ground beef, ground pork, grated Parmesan cheese, almond flour, heavy cream, egg, minced garlic, dried oregano, dried basil, and ground paprika. Mix until well combined.
3. Form the mixture into 1-inch meatballs and place them on a baking sheet lined with parchment paper.
4. Bake in the preheated oven for 20-25 minutes, until the meatballs are cooked through and browned.
5. Serve hot, optionally with a low-carb marinara sauce.

Nutrition Info Per Serving (4 meatballs):
- Calories: 320
- Total Fat: 24g
- Saturated Fat: 10g
- Cholesterol: 100mg
- Sodium: 200mg
- Total Carbohydrates: 3g
- Dietary Fiber: 1g
- Sugars: 0g
- Protein: 22g

Number of Servings: 6
Cooking Time: 25 minutes

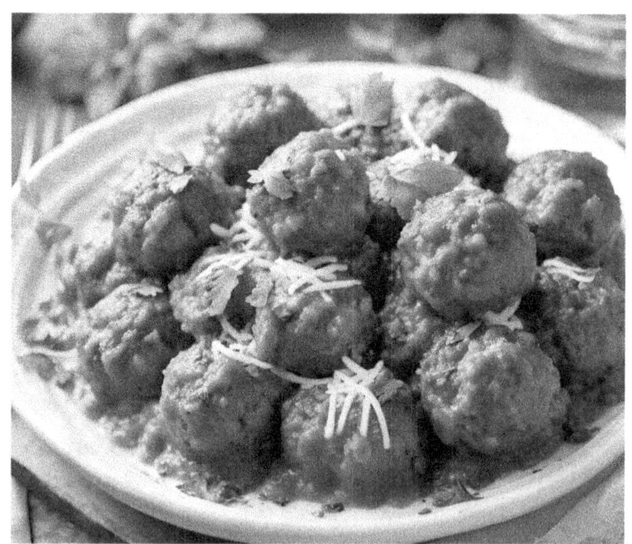

11. Beef and Eggplant Lasagna

Ingredients:

- 1 lb ground beef
- 1 large eggplant, sliced into 1/4-inch rounds
- 1 cup ricotta cheese
- 1 cup shredded mozzarella cheese
- 1/2 cup grated Parmesan cheese
- 1/2 cup heavy cream
- 1 small onion, finely chopped
- 2 cloves garlic, minced
- 1 cup low-carb marinara sauce
- 2 tablespoons olive oil
- 1 tablespoon dried oregano
- 1 tablespoon dried basil

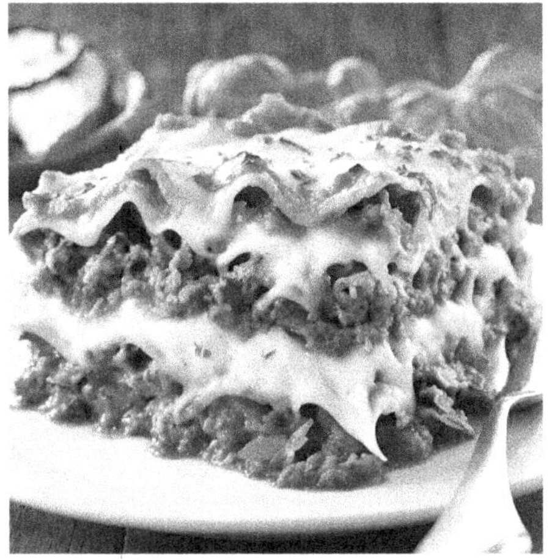

Instructions:

1. Preheat your oven to 375°F (190°C).
2. Heat the olive oil in a large skillet over medium-high heat. Add the chopped onion and cook until translucent, about 3 minutes.
3. Add the minced garlic and ground beef to the skillet. Cook until the beef is browned, breaking it up with a spoon, about 5-7 minutes.
4. Stir in the dried oregano, dried basil, and marinara sauce. Simmer for 5 minutes.
5. In a mixing bowl, combine the ricotta cheese, heavy cream, and half of the grated Parmesan cheese.
6. In a baking dish, layer half of the eggplant slices on the bottom.
7. Spread half of the ricotta mixture over the eggplant slices.
8. Top with half of the meat sauce.
9. Repeat the layers with the remaining eggplant slices, ricotta mixture, and meat sauce.
10. Sprinkle the shredded mozzarella cheese and the remaining grated Parmesan cheese on top.
11. Bake in the preheated oven for 25-30 minutes, until the cheese is melted and bubbly.
12. Let the lasagna rest for 10 minutes before slicing and serving.

Nutrition Info Per Serving (1 slice):

- Calories: 380   Total Fat: 28g   Saturated Fat: 13g   Cholesterol: 90mg
- Sodium: 300mg   Total Carbohydrates: 8g   Dietary Fiber: 3g
- Sugars: 3g
- Protein: 20g

Number of Servings: 6 Cooking Time: 45 minutes

12. Pork Skewers with Satay Sauce

Ingredients:

- 1.5 lbs pork tenderloin, cut into 1-inch cubes
- 1/4 cup coconut milk
- 2 tablespoons soy sauce (or coconut aminos for a soy-free option)
- 2 cloves garlic, minced
- 1 tablespoon grated ginger
- 1 tablespoon olive oil
- 1 teaspoon ground coriander
- 1 teaspoon ground cumin

For the Satay Sauce:

- 1/2 cup full-fat coconut milk
- 1/4 cup natural peanut butter (no sugar added)
- 1 tablespoon soy sauce (or coconut aminos)
- 1 tablespoon lime juice
- 1 teaspoon ground ginger
- 1 teaspoon garlic powder
- 1 teaspoon ground turmeric

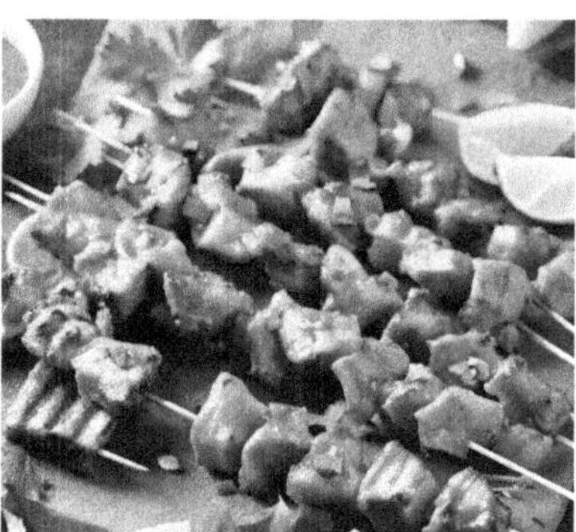

Instructions:

1. In a bowl, combine coconut milk, soy sauce, minced garlic, grated ginger, olive oil, ground coriander, and ground cumin. Mix well.
2. Add the pork cubes to the marinade, cover, and refrigerate for at least 1 hour, or overnight for best results.
3. Preheat the grill to medium-high heat.
4. Thread the marinated pork onto skewers.
5. Grill the skewers for 10-12 minutes, turning occasionally, until the pork is cooked through and slightly charred.
6. While the pork is grilling, prepare the satay sauce by combining all the sauce ingredients in a small saucepan. Cook over medium heat, stirring frequently, until the sauce is smooth and heated through.
7. Serve the pork skewers with the satay sauce on the side.

Nutrition Info Per Serving (2 skewers with sauce):

- Calories: 400   Total Fat: 28g   Saturated Fat: 12g   Cholesterol: 80mg
- Sodium: 400mg   Total Carbohydrates: 6g   Dietary Fiber: 2g   Sugars: 2g
- Protein: 30g

Number of Servings: 4 Cooking Time: 15 minutes (plus marinating time)

13. Keto Chili

Ingredients:

- 1 lb ground beef
- 1 lb ground pork
- 1 cup chopped bell peppers
- 1 small onion, chopped
- 2 cloves garlic, minced
- 1 can (14.5 oz) diced tomatoes (no added sugar)
- 1 can (14.5 oz) tomato sauce (no added sugar)
- 1/4 cup tomato paste
- 2 tablespoons chili powder
- 1 tablespoon ground cumin
- 1 teaspoon paprika
- 1 teaspoon dried oregano
- 2 tablespoons olive oil

Instructions:

1. Heat olive oil in a large pot over medium-high heat.
2. Add the chopped onion and bell peppers to the pot. Cook until softened, about 5 minutes.
3. Add the minced garlic and cook for another 1-2 minutes.
4. Add the ground beef and ground pork to the pot. Cook until browned, breaking up the meat with a spoon, about 7-10 minutes.
5. Stir in the diced tomatoes, tomato sauce, tomato paste, chili powder, ground cumin, paprika, and dried oregano.
6. Bring the chili to a simmer, then reduce the heat to low and cook for 30-45 minutes, stirring occasionally, to allow the flavors to meld.
7. Serve hot, optionally topped with shredded cheese or sour cream.

Nutrition Info Per Serving (1 cup):

- Calories: 450
- Total Fat: 35g
- Saturated Fat: 14g
- Cholesterol: 100mg
- Sodium: 600mg
- Total Carbohydrates: 8g
- Dietary Fiber: 2g
- Sugars: 4g
- Protein: 28g

Number of Servings: 6

Cooking Time: 1 hour

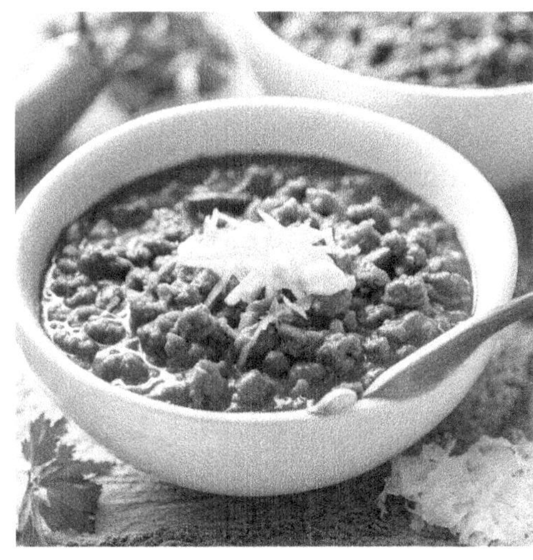

14. German Bratwurst with Sauerkraut

Ingredients:

- 6 bratwurst sausages
- 1 tablespoon olive oil
- 1 small onion, thinly sliced
- 2 cups sauerkraut (drained if necessary)
- 1/2 cup chicken broth
- 1 tablespoon caraway seeds

Instructions:

1. Heat the olive oil in a large skillet over medium-high heat.
2. Add the bratwurst sausages and cook until browned on all sides, about 5-7 minutes. Remove the sausages from the skillet and set aside.
3. In the same skillet, add the sliced onion and cook until softened, about 3-4 minutes.
4. Add the sauerkraut, chicken broth, and caraway seeds to the skillet. Stir well to combine.
5. Return the bratwurst sausages to the skillet, nestling them into the sauerkraut mixture.
6. Reduce the heat to low, cover, and simmer for 20-25 minutes, until the sausages are cooked through and the flavors have melded.
7. Serve hot.

Nutrition Info Per Serving (1 bratwurst with sauerkraut):

- Calories: 350
- Total Fat: 28g
- Saturated Fat: 10g
- Cholesterol: 60mg
- Sodium: 800mg
- Total Carbohydrates: 6g
- Dietary Fiber: 2g
- Sugars: 2g
- Protein: 16g

Number of Servings: 6
Cooking Time: 30 minutes

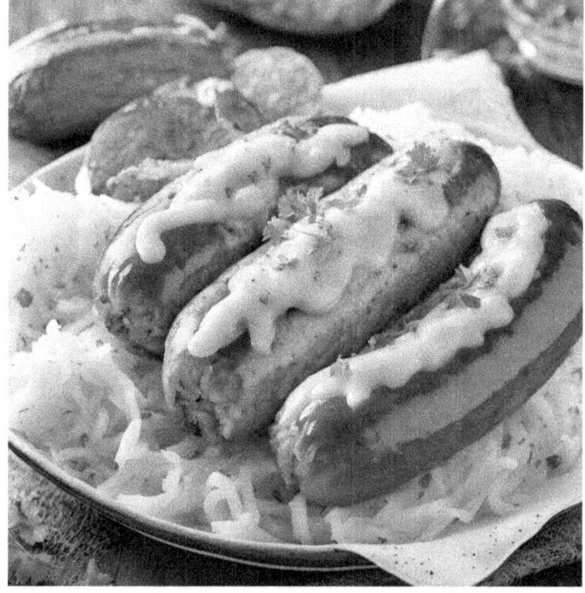

15. Ribeye Steak with Blue Cheese Sauce

Ingredients:

- 4 ribeye steaks (8 oz each)
- 2 tablespoons olive oil
- 1/2 cup heavy cream
- 1/4 cup crumbled blue cheese
- 1 tablespoon butter
- 1 teaspoon garlic powder
- 1 teaspoon dried thyme

Instructions:

1. Preheat your grill or skillet to medium-high heat.
2. Drizzle the olive oil over the ribeye steaks and rub in the garlic powder and dried thyme.
3. Grill or cook the steaks for 4-5 minutes per side for medium-rare, or until they reach your desired level of doneness.
4. While the steaks are cooking, prepare the blue cheese sauce. In a small saucepan, combine the heavy cream, crumbled blue cheese, and butter.
5. Cook over medium heat, stirring frequently, until the cheese is melted and the sauce is smooth, about 5 minutes.
6. Remove the steaks from the grill or skillet and let them rest for 5 minutes.
7. Serve the steaks with the blue cheese sauce drizzled on top.

Nutrition Info Per Serving (1 steak with sauce):

- Calories: 600
- Total Fat: 48g
- Saturated Fat: 20g
- Cholesterol: 160mg
- Sodium: 350mg
- Total Carbohydrates: 2g
- Dietary Fiber: 0g
- Sugars: 1g
- Protein: 38g

Number of Servings: 4
Cooking Time: 20 minutes

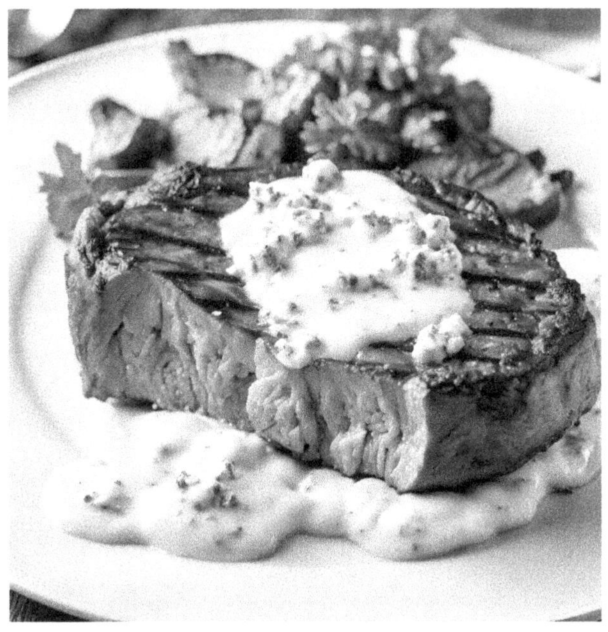

16. Pork Scallopini

Ingredients:

- 1.5 lbs pork tenderloin, sliced into thin medallions
- 1/2 cup almond flour
- 1/4 cup grated Parmesan cheese
- 1/4 cup heavy cream
- 2 tablespoons olive oil
- 2 tablespoons butter
- 1/2 cup chicken broth
- 2 cloves garlic, minced
- 1 tablespoon lemon juice
- 1 tablespoon chopped fresh parsley
- 1 teaspoon dried thyme

Instructions:

1. In a shallow dish, combine the almond flour and grated Parmesan cheese.
2. Dredge each pork medallion in the almond flour mixture, coating both sides.
3. Heat the olive oil and butter in a large skillet over medium-high heat.
4. Add the pork medallions to the skillet and cook for 3-4 minutes per side, until golden brown and cooked through. Remove the pork from the skillet and set aside.
5. In the same skillet, add the minced garlic and sauté for 1 minute.
6. Pour in the chicken broth and lemon juice, stirring to deglaze the pan.
7. Reduce the heat to medium and stir in the heavy cream and dried thyme. Simmer for 2-3 minutes until the sauce thickens.
8. Return the pork medallions to the skillet and coat them with the sauce.
9. Garnish with chopped fresh parsley before serving.

Nutrition Info Per Serving (1 serving):

- Calories: 400
- Total Fat: 28g
- Saturated Fat: 10g
- Cholesterol: 110mg
- Sodium: 320mg
- Total Carbohydrates: 4g
- Dietary Fiber: 1g
- Sugars: 1g
- Protein: 30g

Number of Servings: 4

Cooking Time: 20 minutes

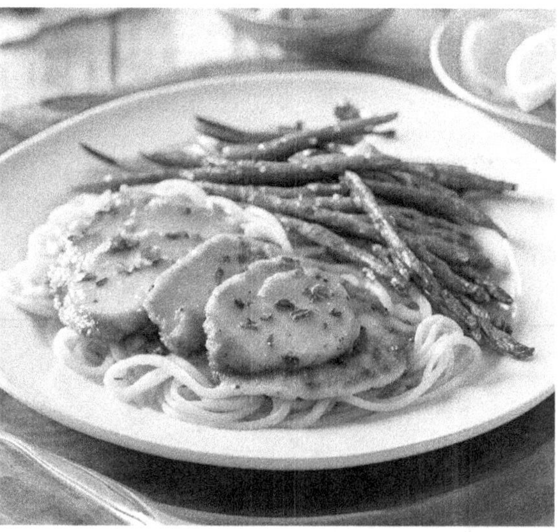

17. Beef Cheek Ragu

Ingredients:

- 2 lbs beef cheeks
- 1 cup beef broth
- 1 cup red wine
- 1 can (14.5 oz) diced tomatoes (no added sugar)
- 1 small onion, chopped
- 2 cloves garlic, minced
- 2 tablespoons tomato paste
- 2 tablespoons olive oil
- 1 tablespoon dried oregano
- 1 tablespoon dried basil
- 1 teaspoon ground paprika

Instructions:

1. Heat the olive oil in a large pot or Dutch oven over medium-high heat.
2. Add the beef cheeks and brown on all sides, about 5-7 minutes. Remove the beef cheeks and set aside.
3. In the same pot, add the chopped onion and cook until softened, about 3 minutes.
4. Add the minced garlic and cook for another 1-2 minutes.
5. Stir in the tomato paste and cook for 1 minute.
6. Pour in the red wine and beef broth, stirring to deglaze the pot.
7. Add the diced tomatoes, dried oregano, dried basil, and ground paprika. Stir well.
8. Return the beef cheeks to the pot, cover, and reduce the heat to low.
9. Simmer for 3-4 hours, until the beef cheeks are tender and the sauce has thickened.
10. Shred the beef cheeks with a fork and stir them back into the sauce.
11. Serve hot.

Nutrition Info Per Serving (1 cup):

- Calories: 450
- Total Fat: 30g
- Saturated Fat: 12g
- Cholesterol: 120mg
- Sodium: 400mg
- Total Carbohydrates: 6g
- Dietary Fiber: 2g
- Sugars: 3g
- Protein: 32g

Number of Servings: 6
Cooking Time: 4 hours

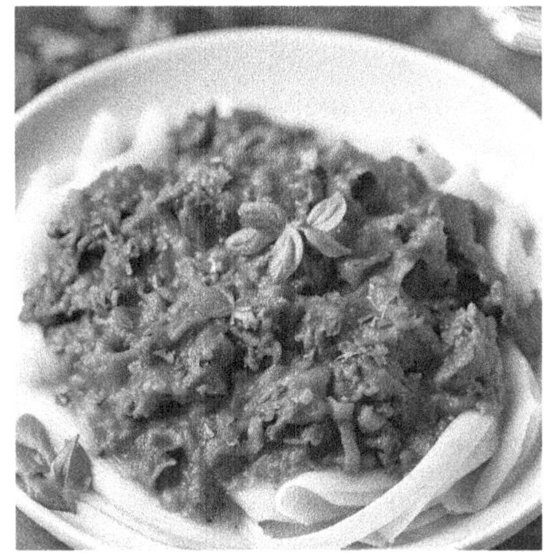

18. Keto Beef Bourguignon
Ingredients:
- 2 lbs beef chuck, cut into 1-inch cubes
- 1 cup red wine
- 1 cup beef broth
- 4 slices bacon, chopped
- 1 cup mushrooms, sliced
- 1 small onion, chopped
- 2 cloves garlic, minced
- 2 tablespoons tomato paste
- 2 tablespoons olive oil
- 1 tablespoon dried thyme
- 1 tablespoon dried rosemary

Instructions:
1. Preheat your oven to 325°F (165°C).
2. Heat the olive oil in a large oven-safe pot or Dutch oven over medium-high heat.
3. Add the chopped bacon and cook until crispy. Remove the bacon and set aside, leaving the rendered fat in the pot.
4. Add the beef cubes to the pot and brown on all sides, about 5-7 minutes. Remove the beef and set aside.
5. In the same pot, add the chopped onion and cook until softened, about 3 minutes.
6. Add the minced garlic and cook for another 1-2 minutes.
7. Stir in the tomato paste and cook for 1 minute.
8. Pour in the red wine and beef broth, stirring to deglaze the pot.
9. Add the sliced mushrooms, dried thyme, and dried rosemary. Stir well.
10. Return the beef and bacon to the pot. Cover and transfer to the preheated oven.
11. Cook for 2.5-3 hours, until the beef is tender and the sauce has thickened.
12. Serve hot.

Nutrition Info Per Serving (1 cup):
- Calories: 480
- Total Fat: 34g
- Saturated Fat: 12g
- Cholesterol: 110mg
- Sodium: 420mg
- Total Carbohydrates: 7g
- Dietary Fiber: 2g
- Sugars: 3g
- Protein: 32g

Number of Servings: 6
Cooking Time: 3 hours

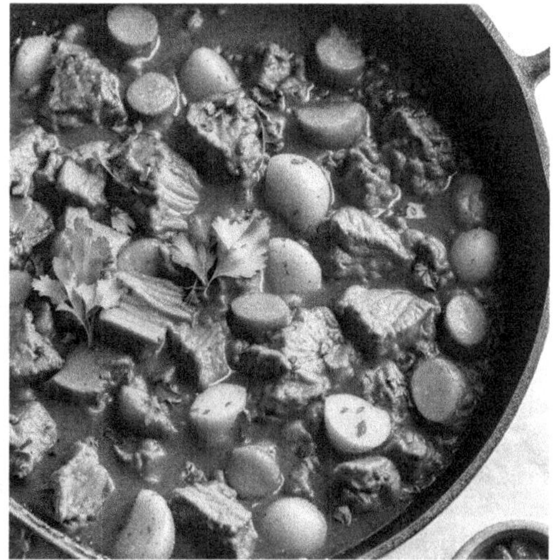

19. Pork and Kimchi Stew

Ingredients:

- 1.5 lbs pork shoulder, cut into 1-inch cubes
- 2 cups kimchi, chopped
- 1 cup kimchi juice
- 1 cup beef broth
- 1 small onion, chopped
- 2 cloves garlic, minced
- 2 tablespoons gochujang (Korean chili paste)
- 1 tablespoon sesame oil
- 1 tablespoon soy sauce (or coconut aminos for a soy-free option)
- 1 teaspoon ground ginger

Instructions:

1. Heat the sesame oil in a large pot over medium-high heat.
2. Add the pork shoulder cubes and brown on all sides, about 5-7 minutes.
3. Add the chopped onion and minced garlic to the pot. Cook until the onion is softened, about 3 minutes.
4. Stir in the gochujang and cook for 1 minute.
5. Add the chopped kimchi, kimchi juice, beef broth, soy sauce, and ground ginger to the pot. Stir well to combine.
6. Bring the stew to a boil, then reduce the heat to low and simmer for 1.5-2 hours, until the pork is tender.
7. Serve hot.

Nutrition Info Per Serving (1 cup):

- Calories: 350
- Total Fat: 24g
- Saturated Fat: 8g
- Cholesterol: 80mg
- Sodium: 800mg
- Total Carbohydrates: 8g
- Dietary Fiber: 2g
- Sugars: 2g
- Protein: 22g

Number of Servings: 6

Cooking Time: 2 hours

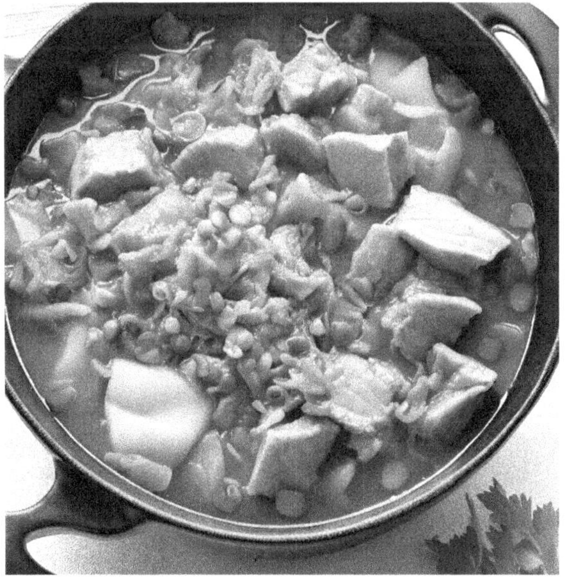

20. Pork Chops with Rosemary and Garlic

Ingredients:

- 4 bone-in pork chops (8 oz each)
- 2 tablespoons olive oil
- 3 cloves garlic, minced
- 2 tablespoons fresh rosemary, chopped
- 1/4 cup heavy cream
- 1/4 cup chicken broth
- 1 tablespoon butter

Instructions:

1. Heat the olive oil in a large skillet over medium-high heat.
2. Add the pork chops and cook for 4-5 minutes per side, until golden brown and cooked through. Remove the pork chops from the skillet and set aside.
3. In the same skillet, add the minced garlic and chopped rosemary. Sauté for 1-2 minutes until fragrant.
4. Add the chicken broth to deglaze the skillet, stirring to incorporate any browned bits from the bottom.
5. Stir in the heavy cream and butter, and cook for 3-4 minutes until the sauce thickens.
6. Return the pork chops to the skillet and coat them with the sauce.
7. Serve immediately.

Nutrition Info Per Serving (1 pork chop with sauce):

- Calories: 420
- Total Fat: 34g
- Saturated Fat: 14g
- Cholesterol: 130mg
- Sodium: 220mg
- Total Carbohydrates: 2g
- Dietary Fiber: 0g
- Sugars: 1g
- Protein: 25g

Number of Servings: 4
Cooking Time: 20 minutes

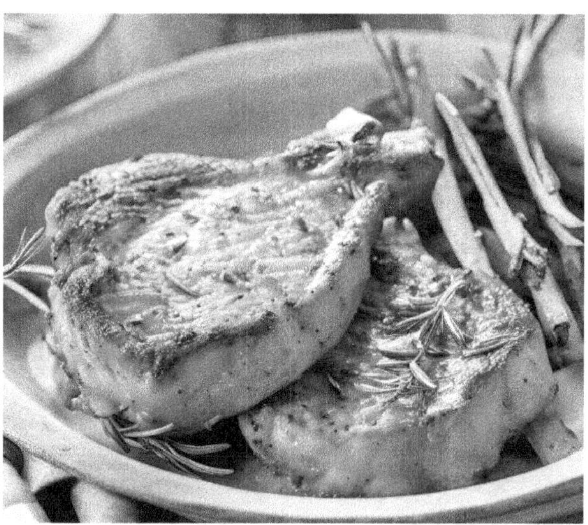

21. Spicy Pork and Zucchini Noodles

Ingredients:

- 1 lb ground pork
- 4 medium zucchinis, spiralized
- 2 tablespoons olive oil
- 1 red bell pepper, sliced
- 3 cloves garlic, minced
- 1 tablespoon soy sauce (or coconut aminos)
- 1 tablespoon sriracha sauce
- 1 teaspoon ground ginger
- 1/2 teaspoon chili flakes
- 2 green onions, chopped

Instructions:

1. Heat 1 tablespoon of olive oil in a large skillet over medium-high heat.
2. Add the ground pork and cook until browned, about 5-7 minutes. Remove the pork from the skillet and set aside.
3. In the same skillet, add the remaining olive oil and minced garlic. Sauté for 1 minute until fragrant.
4. Add the red bell pepper and cook for 3-4 minutes until softened.
5. Stir in the soy sauce, sriracha sauce, ground ginger, and chili flakes. Cook for 1-2 minutes.
6. Add the spiralized zucchini noodles and cooked pork to the skillet. Toss to combine and cook for another 2-3 minutes until the zucchini noodles are tender.
7. Garnish with chopped green onions and serve immediately.

Nutrition Info Per Serving (1 bowl):

- Calories: 320
- Total Fat: 24g
- Saturated Fat: 7g
- Cholesterol: 70mg
- Sodium: 360mg
- Total Carbohydrates: 6g
- Dietary Fiber: 2g
- Sugars: 3g
- Protein: 20g

Number of Servings: 4
Cooking Time: 20 minutes

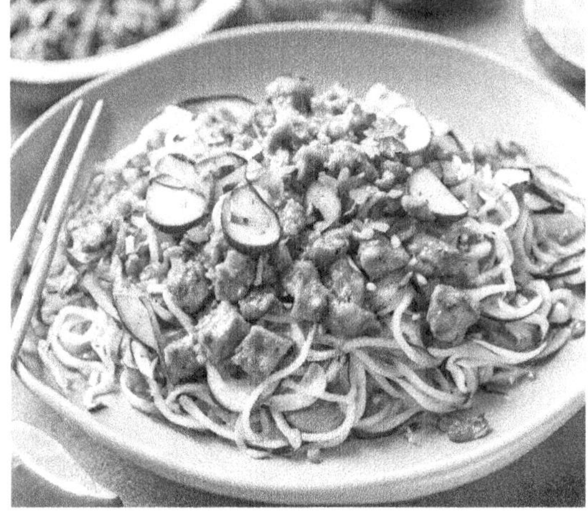

22. Balsamic Glazed Steak Rolls

Ingredients:

- 1 lb flank steak, thinly sliced into strips
- 1/2 cup balsamic vinegar
- 2 tablespoons olive oil
- 1 tablespoon Dijon mustard
- 2 cloves garlic, minced
- 1 red bell pepper, julienned
- 1 yellow bell pepper, julienned
- 1 zucchini, julienned
- 1 tablespoon dried oregano

Instructions:

1. In a small bowl, mix together the balsamic vinegar, olive oil, Dijon mustard, minced garlic, and dried oregano.
2. Place the steak strips in a shallow dish and pour the balsamic marinade over them. Cover and refrigerate for at least 1 hour.
3. Preheat your grill or grill pan to medium-high heat.
4. Remove the steak strips from the marinade and lay them flat. Place a few pieces of red bell pepper, yellow bell pepper, and zucchini at one end of each strip. Roll up the steak strips around the vegetables and secure with toothpicks.
5. Grill the steak rolls for 2-3 minutes per side, until the steak is cooked to your desired level of doneness.
6. Serve immediately.

Nutrition Info Per Serving (2 rolls):

- Calories: 280
- Total Fat: 18g
- Saturated Fat: 4g
- Cholesterol: 50mg
- Sodium: 180mg
- Total Carbohydrates: 5g
- Dietary Fiber: 1g
- Sugars: 3g
- Protein: 22g

Number of Servings: 4
Cooking Time: 15 minutes
(plus marinating time)

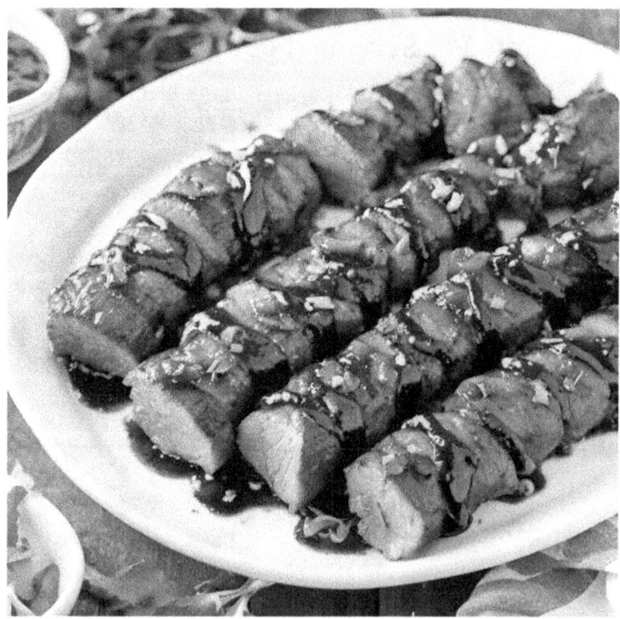

23. Pork Loin Roast with Herb Crust

Ingredients:

- 2 lbs pork loin roast
- 2 tablespoons olive oil
- 3 cloves garlic, minced
- 2 tablespoons fresh rosemary, chopped
- 1 tablespoon fresh thyme, chopped
- 1 tablespoon Dijon mustard
- 1/4 cup grated Parmesan cheese

Instructions:

1. Preheat your oven to 375°F (190°C).
2. In a small bowl, combine the minced garlic, chopped rosemary, chopped thyme, Dijon mustard, grated Parmesan cheese, and olive oil to form a paste.
3. Rub the herb paste evenly over the pork loin roast.
4. Place the pork loin on a rack in a roasting pan.
5. Roast in the preheated oven for 45-50 minutes, or until the internal temperature reaches 145°F (63°C).
6. Remove the pork loin from the oven and let it rest for 10 minutes before slicing.
7. Serve immediately.

Nutrition Info Per Serving (1 slice):

- Calories: 320
- Total Fat: 22g
- Saturated Fat: 7g
- Cholesterol: 90mg
- Sodium: 200mg
- Total Carbohydrates: 2g
- Dietary Fiber: 0g
- Sugars: 0g
- Protein: 26g

Number of Servings: 6

Cooking Time: 50 minutes

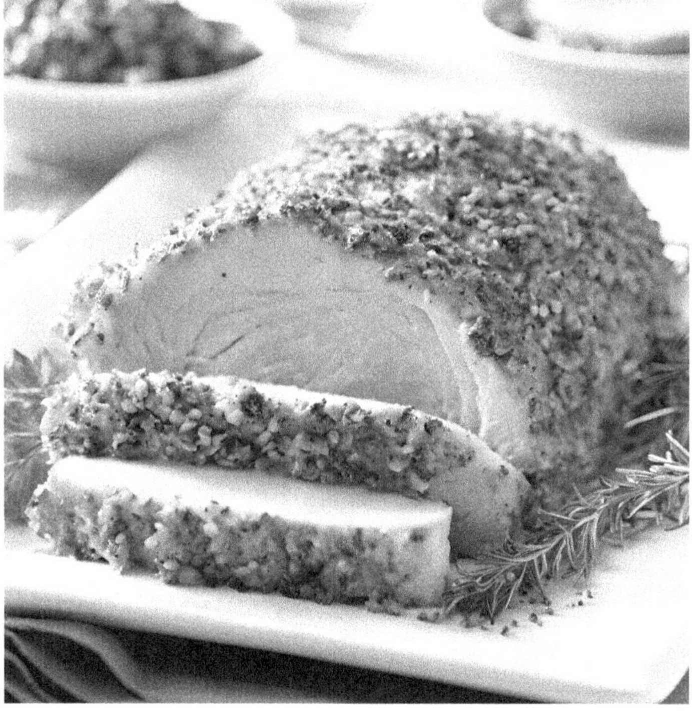

24. Steak and Mushroom Foil Packs

Ingredients:

- 1.5 lbs sirloin steak, cut into bite-sized pieces
- 2 cups sliced mushrooms
- 1 medium onion, sliced
- 3 cloves garlic, minced
- 1/4 cup olive oil
- 2 tablespoons fresh rosemary, chopped
- 1 tablespoon Worcestershire sauce
- 1 teaspoon ground paprika

Instructions:

1. Preheat your grill to medium-high heat.
2. In a large bowl, combine the steak pieces, sliced mushrooms, onion, minced garlic, olive oil, chopped rosemary, Worcestershire sauce, and ground paprika. Mix well.
3. Cut four large pieces of aluminum foil and divide the steak and mushroom mixture evenly among them.
4. Fold the foil over the mixture and seal the edges tightly to form packets.
5. Place the foil packs on the grill and cook for 10-12 minutes, turning halfway through, until the steak is cooked to your desired level of doneness.
6. Remove from the grill and carefully open the foil packs.
7. Serve immediately.

Nutrition Info Per Serving (1 foil pack):

- Calories: 450
- Total Fat: 35g
- Saturated Fat: 10g
- Cholesterol: 90mg
- Sodium: 180mg
- Total Carbohydrates: 5g
- Dietary Fiber: 1g
- Sugars: 2g
- Protein: 30g

Number of Servings: 4

Cooking Time: 15 minutes

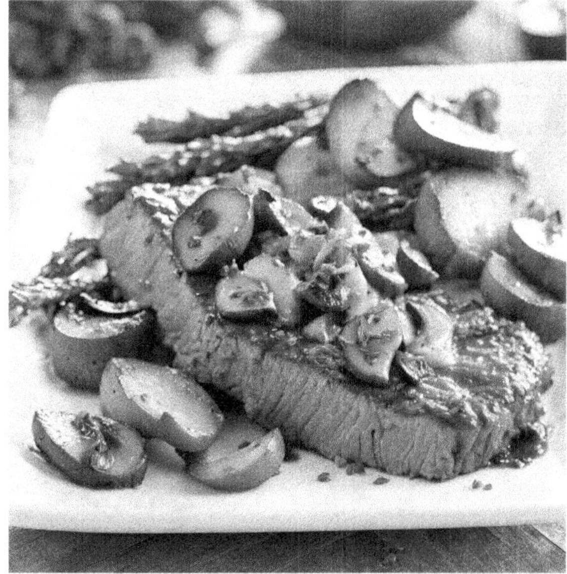

25. Pork Chop with Fennel Salad

Ingredients:

- 4 bone-in pork chops (8 oz each)
- 2 tablespoons olive oil
- 1 teaspoon ground cumin
- 1 teaspoon dried oregano

For the Fennel Salad:

- 2 bulbs fennel, thinly sliced
- 1/4 cup olive oil
- 2 tablespoons lemon juice
- 1 tablespoon Dijon mustard
- 1 teaspoon ground coriander

Instructions:

1. Preheat your grill or skillet to medium-high heat.
2. Rub the pork chops with olive oil, ground cumin, and dried oregano.
3. Grill or cook the pork chops for 4-5 minutes per side, until golden brown and cooked through.
4. While the pork chops are cooking, prepare the fennel salad. In a large bowl, whisk together the olive oil, lemon juice, Dijon mustard, and ground coriander.
5. Add the thinly sliced fennel to the bowl and toss to coat evenly with the dressing.
6. Serve the pork chops with the fennel salad on the side.

Nutrition Info Per Serving (1 pork chop with salad):

- Calories: 500
- Total Fat: 38g
- Saturated Fat: 10g
- Cholesterol: 110mg
- Sodium: 220mg
- Total Carbohydrates: 5g
- Dietary Fiber: 2g
- Sugars: 2g
- Protein: 30g

Number of Servings: 4
Cooking Time: 20 minutes

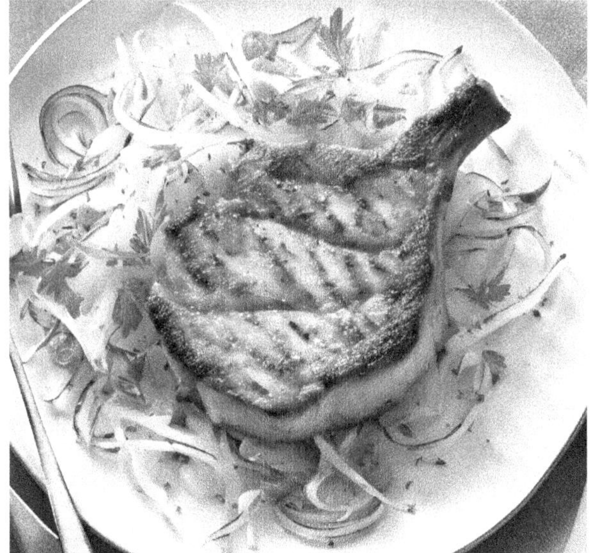

26. Pork and Green Chili

Ingredients:

- 2 lbs pork shoulder, cut into 1-inch cubes
- 1 cup green chili peppers, chopped
- 1 small onion, chopped
- 3 cloves garlic, minced
- 1 cup chicken broth
- 1/2 cup heavy cream
- 2 tablespoons olive oil
- 1 tablespoon ground cumin
- 1 teaspoon dried oregano

Instructions:

1. Heat the olive oil in a large pot over medium-high heat.
2. Add the pork cubes and brown on all sides, about 5-7 minutes. Remove the pork and set aside.
3. In the same pot, add the chopped onion and cook until softened, about 3 minutes.
4. Add the minced garlic and cook for another 1-2 minutes.
5. Stir in the chopped green chili peppers, ground cumin, and dried oregano. Cook for 2 minutes.
6. Return the pork to the pot and add the chicken broth. Bring to a simmer.
7. Reduce the heat to low, cover, and cook for 1.5-2 hours, until the pork is tender.
8. Stir in the heavy cream and cook for an additional 5 minutes.
9. Serve hot.

Nutrition Info Per Serving (1 cup):

- Calories: 450
- Total Fat: 35g
- Saturated Fat: 15g
- Cholesterol: 110mg
- Sodium: 350mg
- Total Carbohydrates: 4g
- Dietary Fiber: 1g
- Sugars: 2g
- Protein: 25g

Number of Servings: 6
Cooking Time: 2 hours

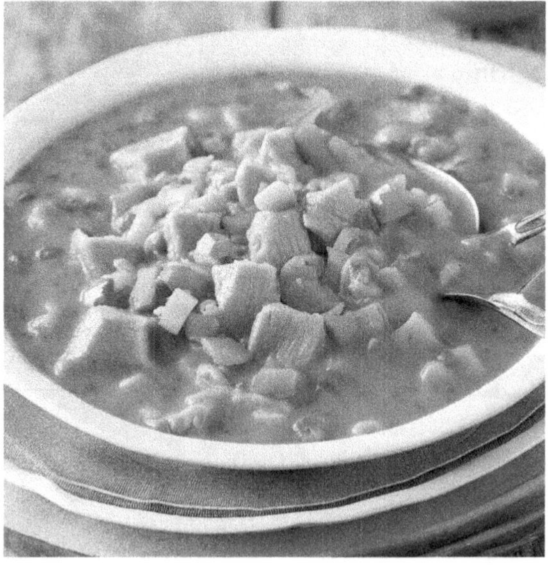

27. Keto Meatloaf

Ingredients:

- 1 lb ground beef
- 1 lb ground pork
- 1/2 cup almond flour
- 1/4 cup grated Parmesan cheese
- 1/2 cup heavy cream
- 1 small onion, finely chopped
- 2 cloves garlic, minced
- 2 large eggs
- 2 tablespoons tomato paste
- 1 tablespoon Worcestershire sauce
- 1 teaspoon dried thyme

Instructions:

1. Preheat your oven to 375°F (190°C).
2. In a large mixing bowl, combine the ground beef, ground pork, almond flour, grated Parmesan cheese, heavy cream, chopped onion, minced garlic, eggs, tomato paste, Worcestershire sauce, and dried thyme. Mix until well combined.
3. Transfer the mixture to a loaf pan and shape it into a loaf.
4. Bake in the preheated oven for 50-60 minutes, until the meatloaf is cooked through and the top is browned.
5. Let the meatloaf rest for 10 minutes before slicing and serving.

Nutrition Info Per Serving (1 slice):

- Calories: 400
- Total Fat: 30g
- Saturated Fat: 12g
- Cholesterol: 120mg
- Sodium: 300mg
- Total Carbohydrates: 5g
- Dietary Fiber: 2g
- Sugars: 2g
- Protein: 25g

Number of Servings: 6
Cooking Time: 1 hour

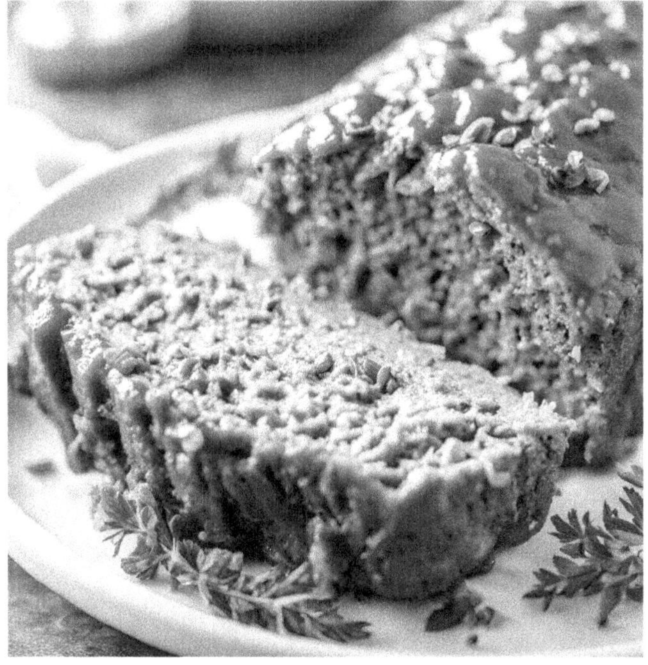

28. Bacon Cheeseburger Casserole

Ingredients:

- 1 lb ground beef
- 8 slices bacon, cooked and crumbled
- 1 cup shredded cheddar cheese
- 4 large eggs
- 1/2 cup heavy cream
- 1 small onion, chopped
- 2 cloves garlic, minced
- 2 tablespoons tomato paste
- 1 tablespoon Dijon mustard
- 1 teaspoon dried oregano

Instructions:

1. Preheat your oven to 350°F (175°C).
2. In a large skillet, cook the ground beef over medium-high heat until browned, about 5-7 minutes. Drain any excess fat.
3. Add the chopped onion and minced garlic to the skillet and cook until softened, about 3 minutes.
4. Stir in the tomato paste, Dijon mustard, and dried oregano. Cook for another 2 minutes.
5. In a large mixing bowl, whisk together the eggs and heavy cream.
6. Transfer the beef mixture to a greased 9x13-inch baking dish.
7. Pour the egg mixture over the beef and top with crumbled bacon and shredded cheddar cheese.
8. Bake in the preheated oven for 25-30 minutes, until the casserole is set and the cheese is melted and bubbly.
9. Let the casserole cool for a few minutes before slicing and serving.

Nutrition Info Per Serving (1 slice):

- Calories: 450
- Total Fat: 35g
- Saturated Fat: 15g
- Cholesterol: 130mg
- Sodium: 380mg
- Total Carbohydrates: 4g
- Dietary Fiber: 1g
- Sugars: 2g
- Protein: 28g

Number of Servings: 6

Cooking Time: 30 minutes

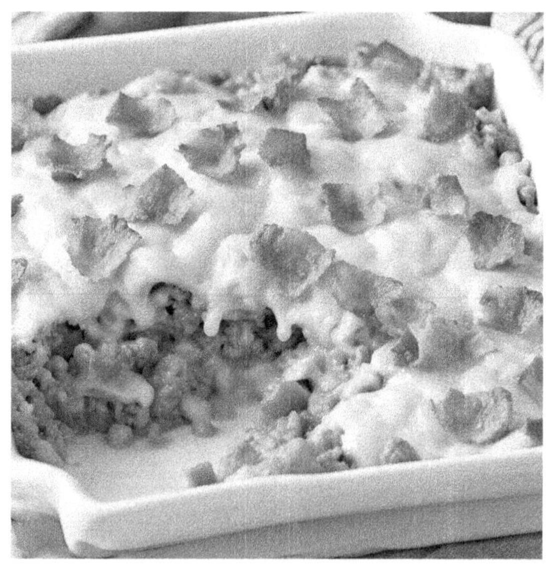

1. Chicken Thighs with Creamy Garlic Sauce

Ingredients:

- 6 bone-in, skin-on chicken thighs
- 2 tablespoons olive oil
- 1 cup heavy cream
- 1/2 cup chicken broth
- 6 cloves garlic, minced
- 1 teaspoon dried thyme
- 1 teaspoon dried rosemary
- 2 tablespoons butter

Instructions:

1. Preheat your oven to 375°F (190°C).
2. Heat the olive oil in a large oven-safe skillet over medium-high heat.
3. Add the chicken thighs, skin-side down, and sear for 5-7 minutes until the skin is crispy and golden. Flip the thighs and sear the other side for an additional 3-4 minutes. Remove the chicken from the skillet and set aside.
4. In the same skillet, add the minced garlic and sauté for 1-2 minutes until fragrant.
5. Pour in the chicken broth and scrape up any browned bits from the bottom of the skillet.
6. Stir in the heavy cream, dried thyme, and dried rosemary. Bring to a simmer and cook for 2-3 minutes until the sauce begins to thicken.
7. Return the chicken thighs to the skillet, skin-side up. Spoon some of the sauce over the thighs.
8. Transfer the skillet to the preheated oven and bake for 25-30 minutes until the chicken is cooked through and the internal temperature reaches 165°F (74°C).
9. Remove from the oven and let rest for a few minutes before serving.

Nutrition Info Per Serving (1 chicken thigh with sauce):

- Calories: 450
- Total Fat: 38g
- Saturated Fat: 15g
- Cholesterol: 120mg
- Sodium: 220mg
- Total Carbohydrates: 2g
- Dietary Fiber: 0g
- Sugars: 1g
- Protein: 22g

Number of Servings: 6

Cooking Time: 40 minutes

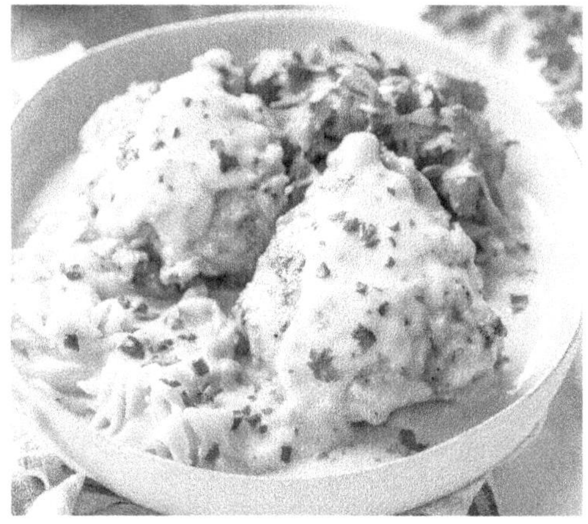

2. Turkey Bacon Wraps

Ingredients:

- 1 lb ground turkey
- 8 slices bacon
- 1/2 cup shredded cheddar cheese
- 1/4 cup mayonnaise (preferably made with avocado oil)
- 1 tablespoon Dijon mustard
- 1 teaspoon dried oregano
- 1 teaspoon garlic powder

Instructions:

1. Preheat your oven to 375°F (190°C).
2. In a mixing bowl, combine the ground turkey, shredded cheddar cheese, mayonnaise, Dijon mustard, dried oregano, and garlic powder. Mix well.
3. Divide the mixture into 8 equal portions and shape them into small patties.
4. Wrap each patty with a slice of bacon and secure with a toothpick.
5. Place the bacon-wrapped turkey patties on a baking sheet lined with parchment paper.
6. Bake in the preheated oven for 20-25 minutes until the bacon is crispy and the turkey is cooked through.
7. Remove from the oven and let rest for a few minutes before serving.

Nutrition Info Per Serving (1 wrap):

- Calories: 300
- Total Fat: 24g
- Saturated Fat: 9g
- Cholesterol: 80mg
- Sodium: 350mg
- Total Carbohydrates: 2g
- Dietary Fiber: 0g
- Sugars: 0g
- Protein: 20g

Number of Servings: 8
Cooking Time: 25 minutes

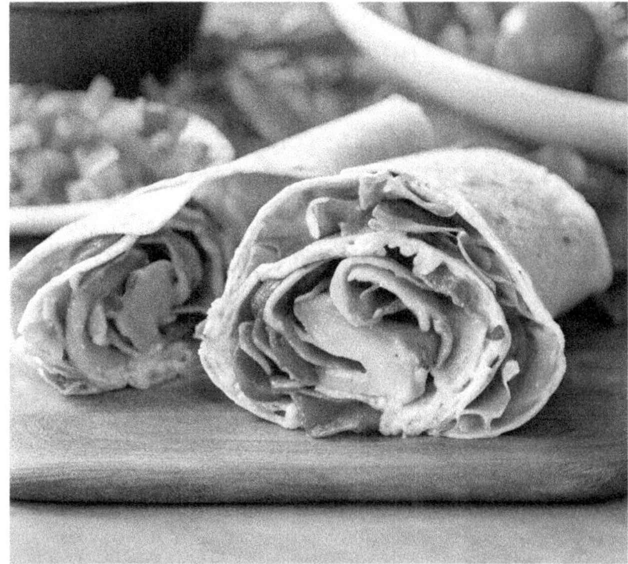

3. Greek Lemon Chicken Soup

Ingredients:

- 1 lb chicken thighs, boneless and skinless, cut into bite-sized pieces
- 6 cups chicken broth
- 1/2 cup heavy cream
- 1/4 cup lemon juice
- 2 eggs
- 1 small onion, chopped
- 2 cloves garlic, minced
- 1 tablespoon olive oil
- 1 teaspoon dried oregano
- 1 teaspoon dried dill

Instructions:

1. Heat the olive oil in a large pot over medium-high heat.
2. Add the chopped onion and cook until softened, about 3 minutes.
3. Add the minced garlic and cook for another 1-2 minutes.
4. Add the chicken pieces to the pot and cook until browned, about 5-7 minutes.
5. Pour in the chicken broth and bring to a simmer. Cook for 10 minutes until the chicken is cooked through.
6. In a small bowl, whisk together the heavy cream, lemon juice, and eggs until smooth.
7. Slowly pour the egg mixture into the soup, stirring constantly to prevent curdling.
8. Stir in the dried oregano and dried dill. Simmer for another 5 minutes until the soup thickens slightly.
9. Serve hot.

Nutrition Info Per Serving (1 cup):

- Calories: 250
- Total Fat: 18g
- Saturated Fat: 8g
- Cholesterol: 120mg
- Sodium: 300mg
- Total Carbohydrates: 3g
- Dietary Fiber: 0g
- Sugars: 1g
- Protein: 20g

Number of Servings: 6

Cooking Time: 30 minutes

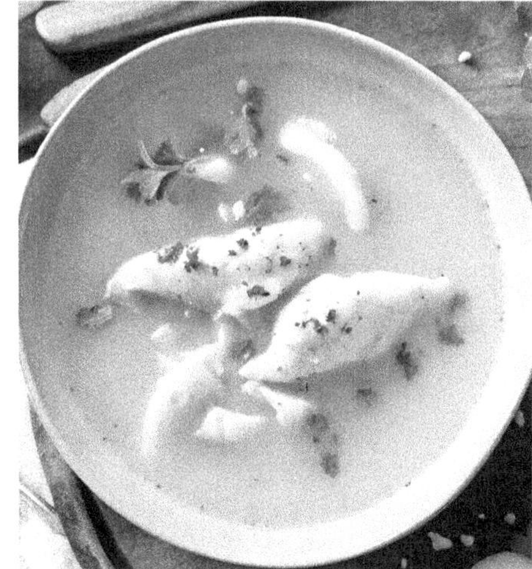

4. Duck Breast with Raspberry Sauce

Ingredients:

- 4 duck breasts
- 1/2 cup fresh raspberries
- 1/4 cup balsamic vinegar
- 1/4 cup chicken broth
- 2 tablespoons butter
- 1 tablespoon honey
- 1 teaspoon dried thyme

Instructions:

1. Preheat your oven to 400°F (200°C).
2. Score the skin of the duck breasts in a crosshatch pattern.
3. Heat a large oven-safe skillet over medium-high heat.
4. Place the duck breasts skin-side down in the skillet and cook for 5-7 minutes until the skin is crispy and golden. Flip the breasts and cook for another 2-3 minutes.
5. Transfer the skillet to the preheated oven and roast for 8-10 minutes until the duck is cooked to your desired level of doneness.
6. Remove the duck breasts from the oven and let rest for 5 minutes.
7. In a small saucepan, combine the raspberries, balsamic vinegar, chicken broth, honey, and dried thyme. Cook over medium heat, stirring frequently, until the sauce thickens and the raspberries break down, about 5 minutes.
8. Stir in the butter until melted and smooth.
9. Slice the duck breasts and serve with the raspberry sauce drizzled over the top.

Nutrition Info Per Serving (1 duck breast with sauce):

- Calories: 450
- Total Fat: 34g
- Saturated Fat: 12g
- Cholesterol: 150mg
- Sodium: 220mg
- Total Carbohydrates: 6g
- Dietary Fiber: 1g
- Sugars: 4g
- Protein: 26g

Number of Servings: 4

Cooking Time: 20 minutes

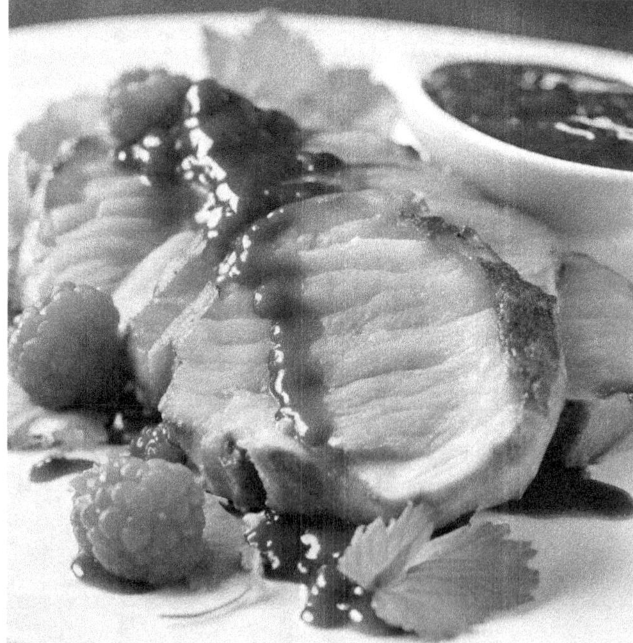

5. Chicken Alfredo with Zucchini Noodles

Ingredients:

- 4 boneless, skinless chicken breasts
- 4 medium zucchinis, spiralized
- 1 cup heavy cream
- 1/2 cup grated Parmesan cheese
- 1/2 cup shredded mozzarella cheese
- 2 cloves garlic, minced
- 2 tablespoons butter
- 2 tablespoons olive oil
- 1 teaspoon dried basil
- 1 teaspoon dried oregano

Instructions:

1. Heat the olive oil in a large skillet over medium-high heat.
2. Add the chicken breasts and cook for 5-7 minutes per side, until golden brown and cooked through. Remove from the skillet and set aside.
3. In the same skillet, melt the butter and sauté the minced garlic for 1-2 minutes until fragrant.
4. Add the heavy cream, grated Parmesan cheese, shredded mozzarella cheese, dried basil, and dried oregano. Stir well to combine and cook until the sauce thickens, about 5 minutes.
5. Slice the cooked chicken breasts and return them to the skillet. Toss to coat with the Alfredo sauce.
6. In a separate skillet, quickly sauté the zucchini noodles for 2-3 minutes until tender.
7. Serve the chicken Alfredo over the zucchini noodles.

Nutrition Info Per Serving (1 serving):

- Calories: 500
- Total Fat: 35g
- Saturated Fat: 18g
- Cholesterol: 160mg
- Sodium: 300mg
- Total Carbohydrates: 6g
- Dietary Fiber: 2g
- Sugars: 3g
- Protein: 40g

Number of Servings: 4

Cooking Time: 20 minutes

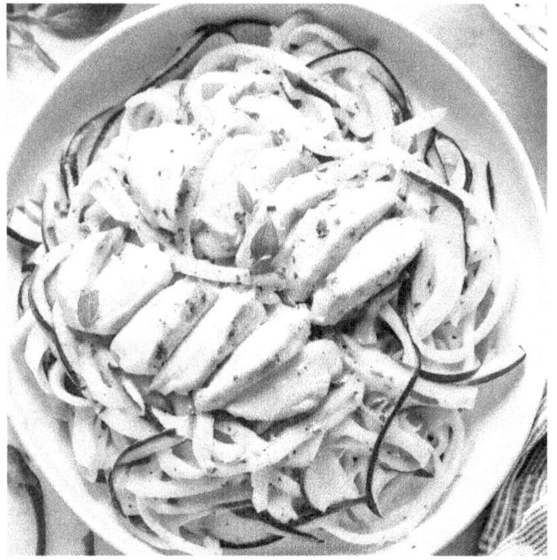

6. Smoked Chicken Wings

Ingredients:

- 2 lbs chicken wings
- 2 tablespoons olive oil
- 1 tablespoon smoked paprika
- 1 teaspoon garlic powder
- 1 teaspoon onion powder
- 1 teaspoon dried thyme

Instructions:

1. Preheat your smoker to 250°F (120°C).
2. In a large bowl, toss the chicken wings with olive oil, smoked paprika, garlic powder, onion powder, and dried thyme until well coated.
3. Arrange the chicken wings on the smoker rack.
4. Smoke the wings for 2-2.5 hours, until they reach an internal temperature of 165°F (74°C) and are crispy on the outside.
5. Remove from the smoker and let rest for a few minutes before serving.

Nutrition Info Per Serving (5 wings):

- Calories: 350
- Total Fat: 28g
- Saturated Fat: 7g
- Cholesterol: 100mg
- Sodium: 240mg
- Total Carbohydrates: 2g
- Dietary Fiber: 0g
- Sugars: 0g
- Protein: 20g

Number of Servings: 4 Cooking Time: 2.5 hours

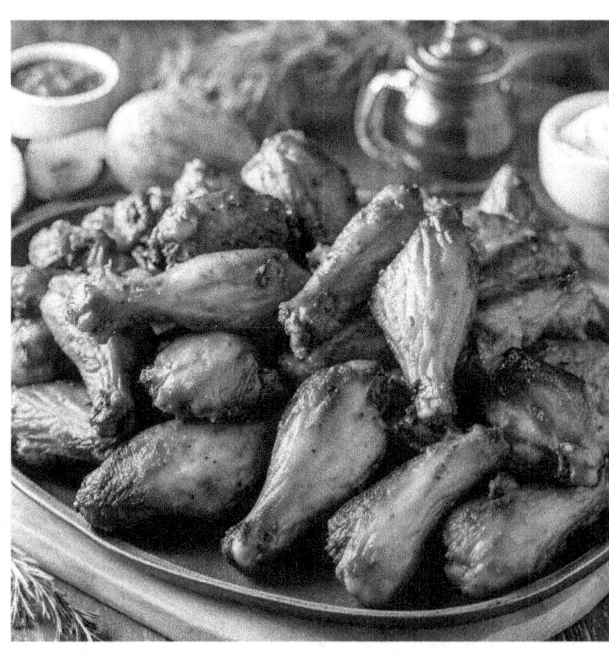

7. Pesto Chicken Casserole

Ingredients:

- 4 boneless, skinless chicken breasts, cut into bite-sized pieces
- 1 cup prepared pesto sauce (preferably homemade or low-carb)
- 1 cup shredded mozzarella cheese
- 1/2 cup grated Parmesan cheese
- 1 cup heavy cream
- 1 tablespoon olive oil
- 1 teaspoon garlic powder
- 1 teaspoon dried basil

Instructions:

1. Preheat your oven to 375°F (190°C).
2. Heat the olive oil in a large skillet over medium-high heat.
3. Add the chicken pieces and cook until browned, about 5-7 minutes. Remove from heat.
4. In a large mixing bowl, combine the pesto sauce, heavy cream, garlic powder, and dried basil. Mix well.
5. Add the cooked chicken to the pesto mixture and stir to coat.
6. Transfer the chicken and pesto mixture to a greased 9x13-inch baking dish.
7. Top with shredded mozzarella and grated Parmesan cheese.
8. Bake in the preheated oven for 20-25 minutes, until the cheese is melted and bubbly.
9. Serve hot.

Nutrition Info Per Serving (1 serving):

- Calories: 550
- Total Fat: 45g
- Saturated Fat: 20g
- Cholesterol: 170mg
- Sodium: 300mg
- Total Carbohydrates: 3g
- Dietary Fiber: 1g
- Sugars: 1g
- Protein: 35g

Number of Servings: 4
Cooking Time: 25 minutes

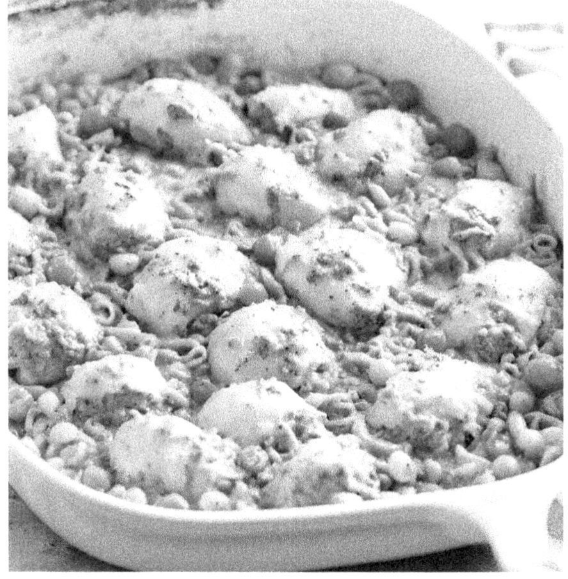

8. Chicken Liver Pâté

Ingredients:

- 1 lb chicken livers, cleaned and trimmed
- 1/2 cup heavy cream
- 1/2 cup butter, divided
- 1 small onion, finely chopped
- 2 cloves garlic, minced
- 1 tablespoon cognac or brandy
- 1 teaspoon dried thyme

Instructions:

1. In a large skillet, melt 1/4 cup of butter over medium heat.
2. Add the chopped onion and minced garlic, and sauté until softened, about 3-4 minutes.
3. Add the chicken livers and cook until browned on the outside and slightly pink on the inside, about 5-7 minutes.
4. Stir in the cognac or brandy and dried thyme. Cook for an additional 2 minutes.
5. Transfer the mixture to a food processor and blend until smooth.
6. Add the heavy cream and the remaining 1/4 cup of butter, blending until fully incorporated.
7. Pour the pâté into a serving dish and refrigerate for at least 2 hours before serving.

Nutrition Info Per Serving (2 tablespoons):

- Calories: 150
- Total Fat: 13g
- Saturated Fat: 7g
- Cholesterol: 90mg
- Sodium: 80mg
- Total Carbohydrates: 1g
- Dietary Fiber: 0g
- Sugars: 0g
- Protein: 8g

Number of Servings: 8
Cooking Time: 15 minutes
(plus 2 hours chilling time)

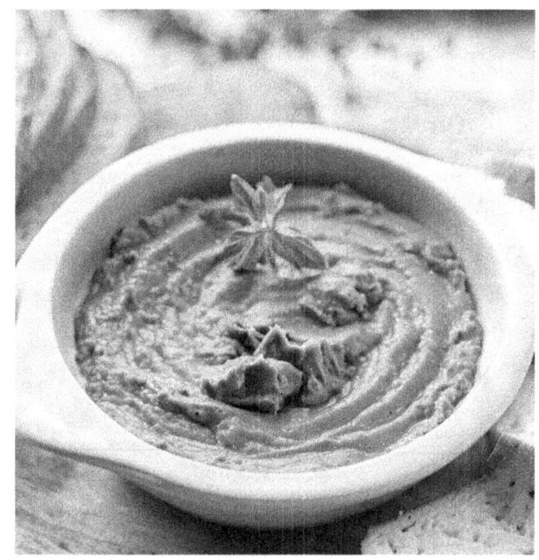

9. Chicken Parmesan (Keto Version)

Ingredients:

- 4 boneless, skinless chicken breasts
- 1 cup almond flour
- 1/2 cup grated Parmesan cheese
- 2 large eggs, beaten
- 1 cup marinara sauce (no added sugar)
- 1 cup shredded mozzarella cheese
- 1/2 cup grated Parmesan cheese
- 1 teaspoon dried oregano
- 1 teaspoon garlic powder
- 1/4 cup olive oil

Instructions:

1. Preheat your oven to 375°F (190°C).
2. In a shallow dish, combine the almond flour, 1/2 cup grated Parmesan cheese, dried oregano, and garlic powder.
3. Dip each chicken breast in the beaten eggs, then coat with the almond flour mixture.
4. Heat the olive oil in a large skillet over medium-high heat.
5. Add the chicken breasts and cook until golden brown on both sides, about 4-5 minutes per side. Remove from heat.
6. Place the chicken breasts in a greased 9x13-inch baking dish.
7. Top each chicken breast with marinara sauce, shredded mozzarella, and the remaining grated Parmesan cheese.
8. Bake in the preheated oven for 20-25 minutes, until the cheese is melted and bubbly.
9. Serve hot.

Nutrition Info Per Serving (1 chicken breast with sauce and cheese):

- Calories: 450
- Total Fat: 30g
- Saturated Fat: 10g
- Cholesterol: 150mg
- Sodium: 400mg
- Total Carbohydrates: 6g
- Dietary Fiber: 2g
- Sugars: 2g
- Protein: 35g

Number of Servings: 4
Cooking Time: 30 minutes

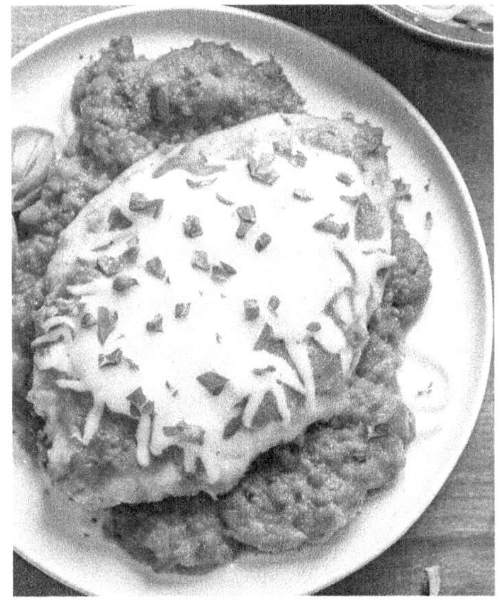

10. Roasted Quail with Herbs

Ingredients:

- 6 quail
- 1/4 cup olive oil
- 2 tablespoons butter, melted
- 2 tablespoons fresh rosemary, chopped
- 2 tablespoons fresh thyme, chopped
- 4 cloves garlic, minced
- 1 lemon, sliced

Instructions:

1. Preheat your oven to 400°F (200°C).
2. In a small bowl, mix together the olive oil, melted butter, chopped rosemary, chopped thyme, and minced garlic.
3. Rub the herb mixture all over the quail.
4. Place the quail in a roasting pan and arrange the lemon slices around them.
5. Roast in the preheated oven for 25-30 minutes, until the quail are golden brown and cooked through.
6. Let rest for 5 minutes before serving.

Nutrition Info Per Serving (1 quail):

- Calories: 320
- Total Fat: 24g
- Saturated Fat: 7g
- Cholesterol: 100mg
- Sodium: 140mg
- Total Carbohydrates: 1g
- Dietary Fiber: 0g
- Sugars: 0g
- Protein: 22g

Number of Servings: 6 Cooking Time: 30 minutes

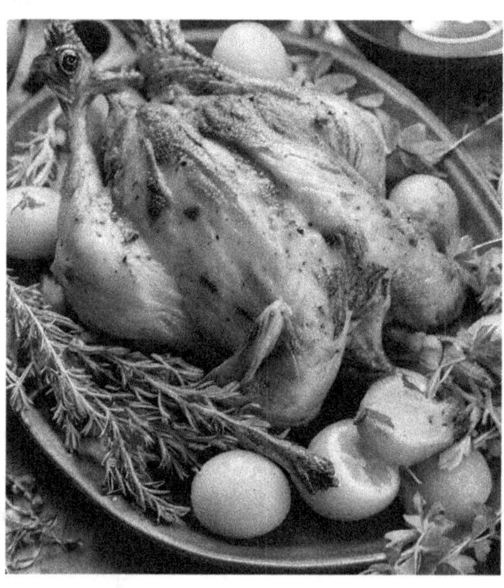

11. Chicken Skewers with Tzatziki Sauce

Ingredients:

- 2 lbs boneless, skinless chicken thighs, cut into bite-sized pieces
- 1/4 cup olive oil
- 2 tablespoons lemon juice
- 2 cloves garlic, minced
- 1 tablespoon dried oregano

For the Tzatziki Sauce:

- 1 cup full-fat Greek yogurt
- 1 cucumber, grated and squeezed to remove excess water
- 2 cloves garlic, minced
- 1 tablespoon lemon juice
- 1 tablespoon olive oil
- 1 teaspoon dried dill

Instructions:

1. In a large bowl, combine the olive oil, lemon juice, minced garlic, and dried oregano. Add the chicken pieces and toss to coat. Marinate for at least 30 minutes.
2. Preheat your grill or grill pan to medium-high heat.
3. Thread the marinated chicken pieces onto skewers.
4. Grill the chicken skewers for 10-12 minutes, turning occasionally, until the chicken is cooked through.
5. While the chicken is grilling, prepare the tzatziki sauce. In a bowl, mix together the Greek yogurt, grated cucumber, minced garlic, lemon juice, olive oil, and dried dill.
6. Serve the chicken skewers with the tzatziki sauce.

Nutrition Info Per Serving (1 skewer with sauce):

- Calories: 350
- Total Fat: 25g
- Saturated Fat: 8g
- Cholesterol: 120mg
- Sodium: 180mg
- Total Carbohydrates: 3g
- Dietary Fiber: 0g
- Sugars: 1g
- Protein: 25g

Number of Servings: 6

Cooking Time: 15 minutes (plus marinating time)

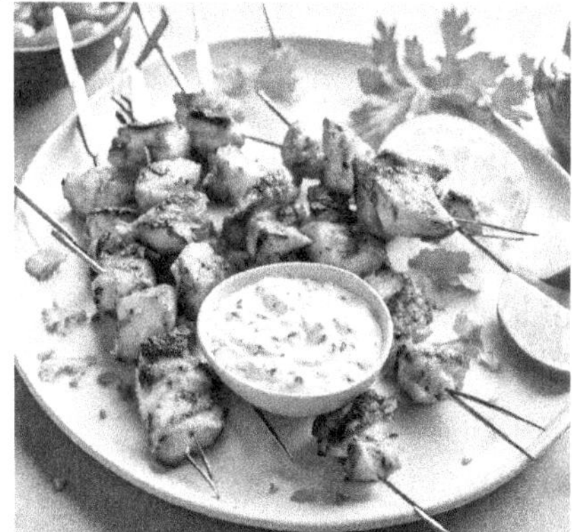

12. Turkey Meatballs in Marinara Sauce

Ingredients:

- 1 lb ground turkey
- 1/4 cup grated Parmesan cheese
- 1/4 cup almond flour
- 1/4 cup heavy cream
- 1 egg
- 2 cloves garlic, minced
- 1 teaspoon dried oregano

For the Marinara Sauce:

- 1 can (14.5 oz) diced tomatoes (no added sugar)
- 1/2 cup tomato sauce (no added sugar)
- 2 cloves garlic, minced
- 1 tablespoon olive oil
- 1 teaspoon dried basil

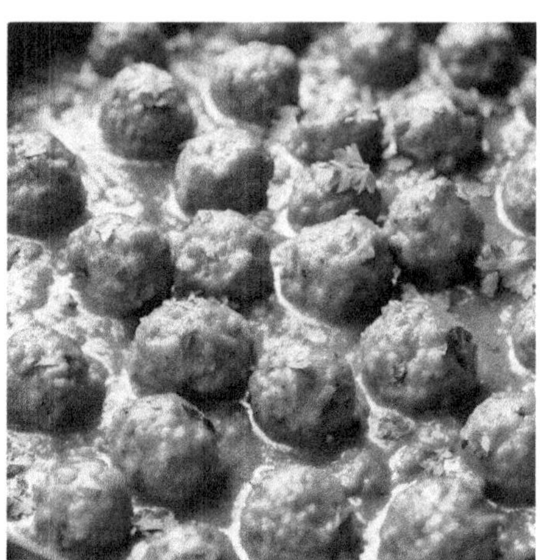

Instructions:

1. Preheat your oven to 375°F (190°C).
2. In a large bowl, combine the ground turkey, grated Parmesan cheese, almond flour, heavy cream, egg, minced garlic, and dried oregano. Mix until well combined.
3. Form the mixture into 1-inch meatballs and place them on a baking sheet lined with parchment paper.
4. Bake in the preheated oven for 20-25 minutes, until the meatballs are cooked through and browned.
5. While the meatballs are baking, prepare the marinara sauce. In a saucepan, heat the olive oil over medium heat.
6. Add the minced garlic and sauté for 1-2 minutes until fragrant.
7. Stir in the diced tomatoes, tomato sauce, and dried basil. Simmer for 10 minutes.
8. Add the baked meatballs to the marinara sauce and simmer for an additional 5 minutes.
9. Serve hot.

Nutrition Info Per Serving (4 meatballs with sauce):

- Calories: 350
- Total Fat: 25g
- Saturated Fat: 10g
- Cholesterol: 120mg
- Sodium: 320mg
- Total Carbohydrates: 6g
- Dietary Fiber: 2g
- Sugars: 3g
- Protein: 22g

Number of Servings: 4 Cooking Time: 35 minutes

13. Mustard Roasted Chicken Thighs

Ingredients:

- 6 bone-in, skin-on chicken thighs
- 1/4 cup Dijon mustard
- 1/4 cup olive oil
- 2 cloves garlic, minced
- 1 tablespoon fresh thyme, chopped
- 1 tablespoon fresh rosemary, chopped

Instructions:

1. Preheat your oven to 400°F (200°C).
2. In a small bowl, mix together the Dijon mustard, olive oil, minced garlic, chopped thyme, and chopped rosemary.
3. Rub the mustard mixture all over the chicken thighs.
4. Place the chicken thighs in a roasting pan.
5. Roast in the preheated oven for 35-40 minutes, until the chicken is golden brown and cooked through.
6. Let rest for 5 minutes before serving.

Nutrition Info Per Serving (1 chicken thigh):

- Calories: 350
- Total Fat: 28g
- Saturated Fat: 8g
- Cholesterol: 100mg
- Sodium: 140mg
- Total Carbohydrates: 2g
- Dietary Fiber: 0g
- Sugars: 0g
- Protein: 22g

Number of Servings: 6 Cooking Time: 40 minutes

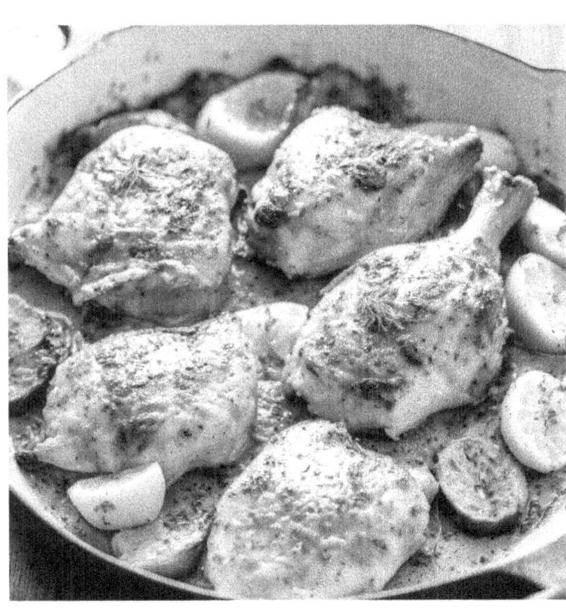

14. Garlic Butter Turkey Meatballs
Ingredients:

- 1 lb ground turkey
- 1/4 cup grated Parmesan cheese
- 1/4 cup almond flour
- 1/4 cup heavy cream
- 1 egg
- 2 cloves garlic, minced
- 1 teaspoon dried oregano

For the Garlic Butter Sauce:

- 1/4 cup butter
- 2 cloves garlic, minced
- 1 tablespoon fresh parsley, chopped

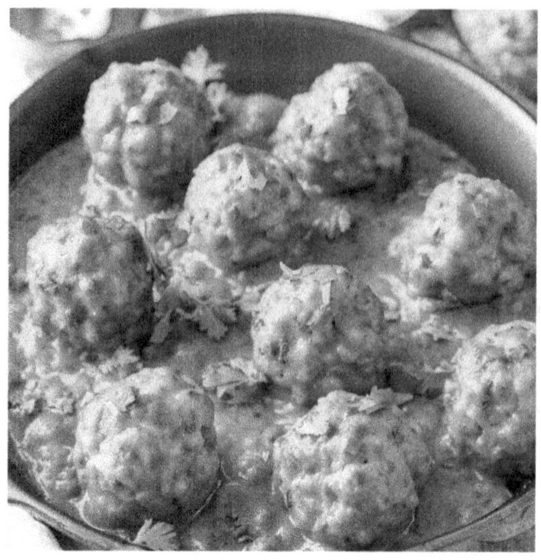

Instructions:

1. Preheat your oven to 375°F (190°C).
2. In a large bowl, combine the ground turkey, grated Parmesan cheese, almond flour, heavy cream, egg, minced garlic, and dried oregano. Mix until well combined.
3. Form the mixture into 1-inch meatballs and place them on a baking sheet lined with parchment paper.
4. Bake in the preheated oven for 20-25 minutes, until the meatballs are cooked through and browned.
5. While the meatballs are baking, prepare the garlic butter sauce. In a saucepan, melt the butter over medium heat.
6. Add the minced garlic and sauté for 1-2 minutes until fragrant.
7. Stir in the chopped parsley and cook for an additional 1 minute.
8. Remove the meatballs from the oven and toss them in the garlic butter sauce.
9. Serve hot.

Nutrition Info Per Serving (4 meatballs with sauce):

- Calories: 320
- Total Fat: 25g
- Saturated Fat: 12g
- Cholesterol: 110mg
- Sodium: 200mg
- Total Carbohydrates: 3g
- Dietary Fiber: 1g
- Sugars: 0g
- Protein: 20g

Number of Servings: 4
Cooking Time: 30 minutes

15. Sesame Chicken Stir-Fry
Ingredients:
- 1.5 lbs boneless, skinless chicken thighs, cut into bite-sized pieces
- 2 tablespoons sesame oil
- 1/4 cup soy sauce (or coconut aminos)
- 2 tablespoons rice vinegar
- 1 tablespoon sesame seeds
- 1 tablespoon grated ginger
- 3 cloves garlic, minced
- 1 red bell pepper, sliced
- 1 cup broccoli florets
- 1/2 cup chopped green onions

Instructions:
1. In a small bowl, whisk together the soy sauce, rice vinegar, grated ginger, and minced garlic.
2. Heat the sesame oil in a large skillet or wok over medium-high heat.
3. Add the chicken pieces and cook until browned and cooked through, about 5-7 minutes.
4. Remove the chicken from the skillet and set aside.
5. In the same skillet, add the red bell pepper and broccoli florets. Stir-fry for 3-4 minutes until tender-crisp.
6. Return the chicken to the skillet and pour the soy sauce mixture over the top. Stir well to coat everything evenly.
7. Cook for another 2-3 minutes until the sauce has thickened slightly.
8. Sprinkle with sesame seeds and chopped green onions before serving.

Nutrition Info Per Serving (1 cup):
- Calories: 350
- Total Fat: 22g
- Saturated Fat: 5g
- Cholesterol: 110mg
- Sodium: 480mg
- Total Carbohydrates: 7g
- Dietary Fiber: 2g
- Sugars: 3g
- Protein: 28g

Number of Servings: 4
Cooking Time: 20 minutes

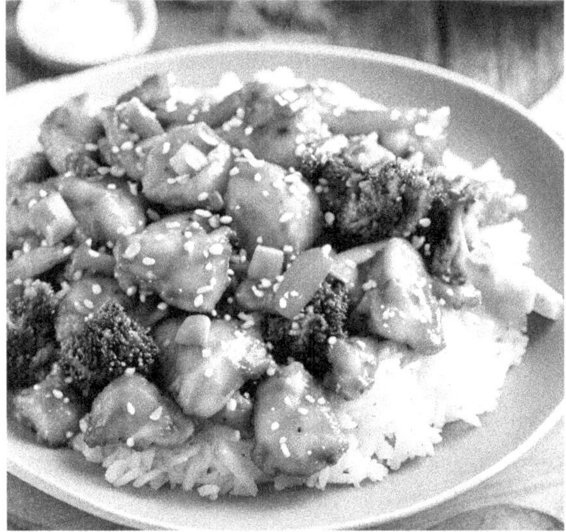

16. Chicken Tikka Masala

Ingredients:

- 1.5 lbs boneless, skinless chicken thighs, cut into bite-sized pieces
- 1 cup full-fat Greek yogurt
- 2 tablespoons lemon juice
- 2 tablespoons garam masala
- 1 tablespoon ground cumin
- 1 tablespoon ground coriander
- 1 tablespoon grated ginger
- 3 cloves garlic, minced
- 1 cup heavy cream
- 1 can (14.5 oz) diced tomatoes (no added sugar)
- 1/2 cup tomato sauce (no added sugar)
- 1 small onion, chopped
- 2 tablespoons ghee (clarified butter)
- 1 teaspoon turmeric
- 1 teaspoon paprika

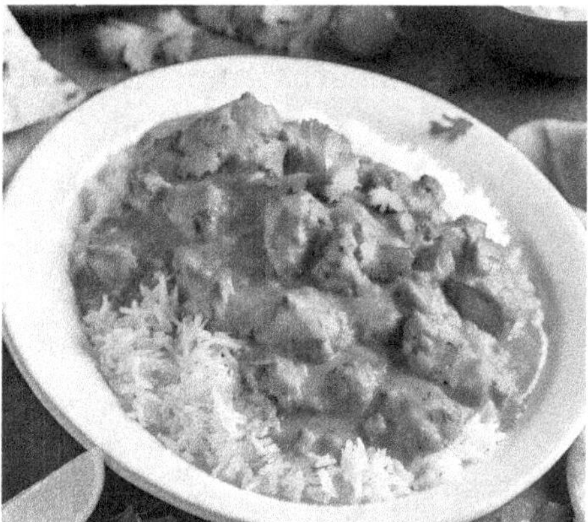

Instructions:

1. In a large bowl, combine the Greek yogurt, lemon juice, garam masala, ground cumin, ground coriander, grated ginger, and minced garlic. Add the chicken pieces and toss to coat. Marinate in the refrigerator for at least 1 hour.
2. Heat the ghee in a large skillet over medium-high heat. Add the chopped onion and sauté until softened, about 3-4 minutes.
3. Add the marinated chicken pieces and cook until browned, about 5-7 minutes.
4. Stir in the turmeric and paprika, and cook for another 1-2 minutes.
5. Add the diced tomatoes and tomato sauce, and bring to a simmer. Cook for 10 minutes.
6. Stir in the heavy cream and simmer for another 5 minutes until the sauce is thickened and the chicken is cooked through.
7. Serve hot.

Nutrition Info Per Serving (1 cup):

- Calories: 450   Total Fat: 32g   Saturated Fat: 18g   Cholesterol: 120mg
- Sodium: 320mg
- Total Carbohydrates: 9g
- Dietary Fiber: 2g
- Sugars: 4g
- Protein: 28g

Number of Servings: 4 Cooking Time: 25 minutes (plus marinating time)

17. Chicken and Mushroom Florentine

Ingredients:

- 4 boneless, skinless chicken breasts
- 2 tablespoons olive oil
- 1/4 cup butter
- 1 small onion, finely chopped
- 2 cloves garlic, minced
- 1 cup sliced mushrooms
- 1 cup heavy cream
- 1/2 cup grated Parmesan cheese
- 1 cup baby spinach

Instructions:

1. Heat the olive oil in a large skillet over medium-high heat.
2. Add the chicken breasts and cook for 5-7 minutes per side, until golden brown and cooked through. Remove from the skillet and set aside.
3. In the same skillet, melt the butter and sauté the chopped onion and minced garlic for 2-3 minutes until fragrant.
4. Add the sliced mushrooms and cook for another 3-4 minutes until tender.
5. Stir in the heavy cream and grated Parmesan cheese. Cook for 3-4 minutes until the sauce thickens.
6. Add the baby spinach and cook until wilted, about 1-2 minutes.
7. Return the chicken breasts to the skillet and coat them with the sauce.
8. Serve hot.

Nutrition Info Per Serving (1 chicken breast with sauce):

- Calories: 500
- Total Fat: 38g
- Saturated Fat: 18g
- Cholesterol: 140mg
- Sodium: 320mg
- Total Carbohydrates: 5g
- Dietary Fiber: 1g
- Sugars: 2g
- Protein: 32g

Number of Servings: 4
Cooking Time: 25 minutes

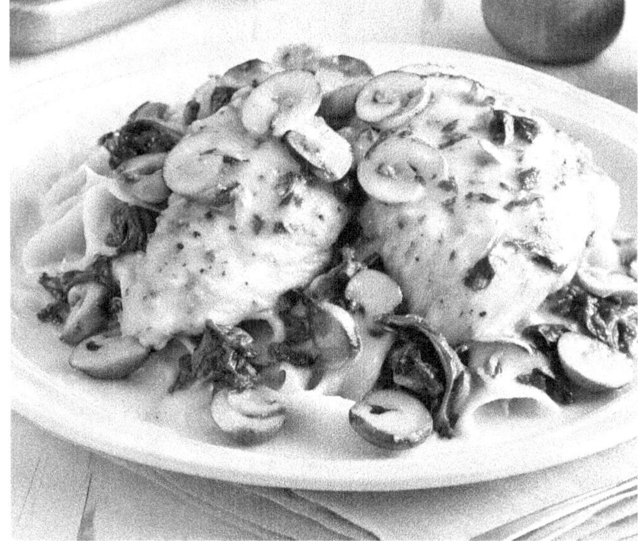

18. Spinach and Feta Stuffed Chicken

Ingredients:

- 4 boneless, skinless chicken breasts
- 1 cup fresh spinach, chopped
- 1/2 cup crumbled feta cheese
- 1/4 cup cream cheese, softened
- 1 tablespoon olive oil
- 2 cloves garlic, minced
- 1 teaspoon dried oregano

Instructions:

1. Preheat your oven to 375°F (190°C).
2. In a mixing bowl, combine the chopped spinach, crumbled feta cheese, softened cream cheese, minced garlic, and dried oregano.
3. Cut a pocket into each chicken breast and stuff with the spinach and feta mixture. Secure with toothpicks if necessary.
4. Heat the olive oil in a large oven-safe skillet over medium-high heat.
5. Add the stuffed chicken breasts and cook for 3-4 minutes per side until golden brown.
6. Transfer the skillet to the preheated oven and bake for 20-25 minutes until the chicken is cooked through.
7. Remove the toothpicks before serving.

Nutrition Info Per Serving (1 stuffed chicken breast):

- Calories: 400
- Total Fat: 28g
- Saturated Fat: 12g
- Cholesterol: 120mg
- Sodium: 320mg
- Total Carbohydrates: 3g
- Dietary Fiber: 1g
- Sugars: 1g
- Protein: 32g

Number of Servings: 4
Cooking Time: 30 minutes

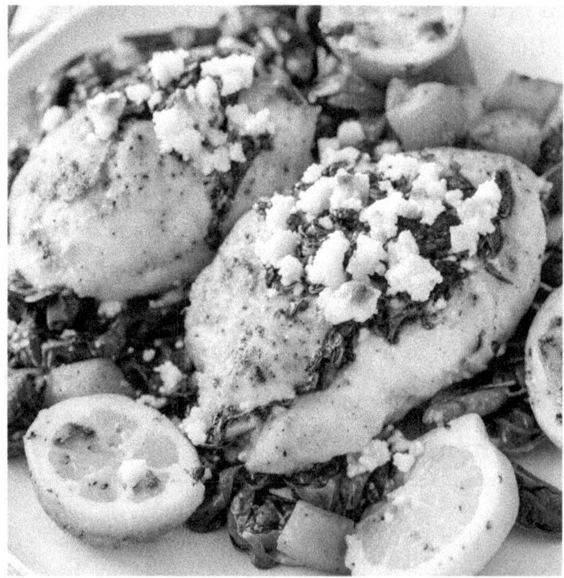

19. Shawarma-Style Chicken

Ingredients:

- 2 lbs boneless, skinless chicken thighs
- 1/4 cup olive oil
- 2 tablespoons lemon juice
- 4 cloves garlic, minced
- 2 teaspoons ground cumin
- 2 teaspoons ground paprika
- 1 teaspoon ground coriander
- 1 teaspoon ground turmeric
- 1 teaspoon ground cinnamon
- 1 teaspoon ground allspice

Instructions:

1. In a large bowl, combine the olive oil, lemon juice, minced garlic, ground cumin, paprika, coriander, turmeric, cinnamon, and allspice. Mix well.
2. Add the chicken thighs to the bowl and toss to coat evenly with the marinade. Cover and refrigerate for at least 1 hour, or overnight for best results.
3. Preheat your grill or grill pan to medium-high heat.
4. Grill the chicken thighs for 5-7 minutes per side, until fully cooked and slightly charred.
5. Remove from the grill and let rest for a few minutes before slicing.
6. Serve hot, optionally with a side of low-carb vegetables or a salad.

Nutrition Info Per Serving (1 chicken thigh):

- Calories: 320
- Total Fat: 22g
- Saturated Fat: 5g
- Cholesterol: 110mg
- Sodium: 100mg
- Total Carbohydrates: 2g
- Dietary Fiber: 1g
- Sugars: 0g
- Protein: 24g

Number of Servings: 6
Cooking Time: 15 minutes
(plus marinating time)

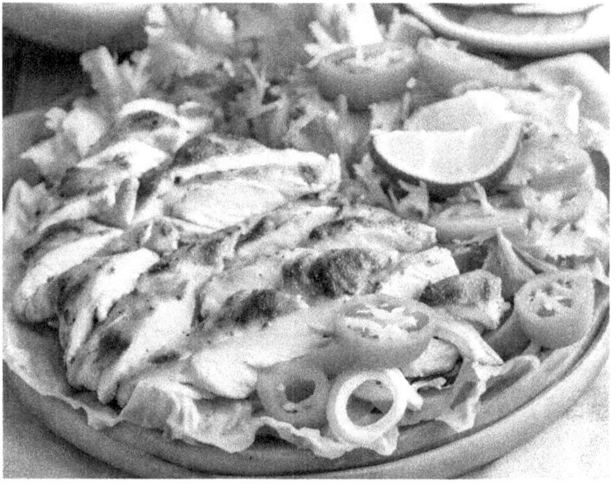

20. Fried Chicken (Almond Flour)

Ingredients:

- 4 boneless, skinless chicken breasts
- 1 cup almond flour
- 1/4 cup grated Parmesan cheese
- 1 teaspoon garlic powder
- 1 teaspoon paprika
- 1 teaspoon dried oregano
- 2 large eggs
- 1/4 cup heavy cream
- 1/4 cup coconut oil (or other high-heat oil) for frying

Instructions:

1. In a shallow dish, combine the almond flour, grated Parmesan cheese, garlic powder, paprika, and dried oregano.
2. In another bowl, whisk together the eggs and heavy cream.
3. Dip each chicken breast into the egg mixture, then coat with the almond flour mixture.
4. Heat the coconut oil in a large skillet over medium-high heat.
5. Fry the chicken breasts for 5-7 minutes per side, until golden brown and cooked through.
6. Remove from the skillet and let rest on a paper towel-lined plate for a few minutes before serving.

Nutrition Info Per Serving (1 fried chicken breast):

- Calories: 450
- Total Fat: 30g
- Saturated Fat: 10g
- Cholesterol: 150mg
- Sodium: 250mg
- Total Carbohydrates: 6g
- Dietary Fiber: 2g
- Sugars: 1g
- Protein: 38g

Number of Servings: 4
Cooking Time: 20 minutes

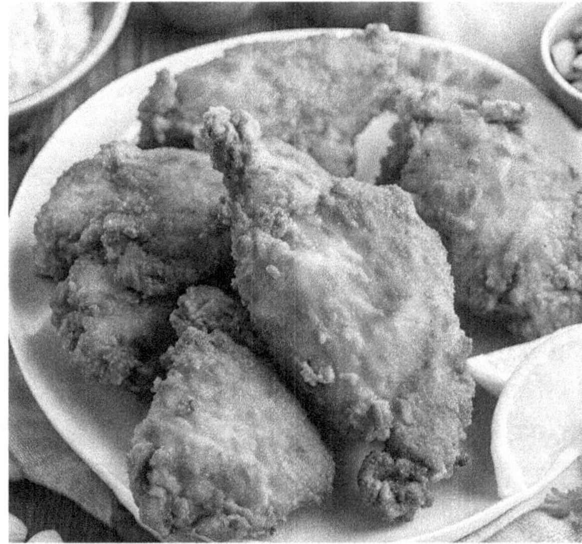

21. Balsamic Glazed Chicken

Ingredients:

- 4 boneless, skinless chicken breasts
- 1/4 cup balsamic vinegar
- 2 tablespoons olive oil
- 1 tablespoon Dijon mustard
- 3 cloves garlic, minced
- 1 tablespoon fresh rosemary, chopped

Instructions:

1. In a small bowl, whisk together the balsamic vinegar, olive oil, Dijon mustard, minced garlic, and chopped rosemary.
2. Place the chicken breasts in a shallow dish and pour the balsamic marinade over them. Cover and refrigerate for at least 30 minutes.
3. Preheat your oven to 375°F (190°C).
4. Heat a large oven-safe skillet over medium-high heat. Add the marinated chicken breasts and sear for 2-3 minutes per side until browned.
5. Transfer the skillet to the preheated oven and bake for 20-25 minutes until the chicken is cooked through.
6. Remove the chicken from the oven and let rest for a few minutes before serving.
7. Drizzle any remaining balsamic glaze from the skillet over the chicken before serving.

Nutrition Info Per Serving (1 chicken breast):

- Calories: 320
- Total Fat: 18g
- Saturated Fat: 4g
- Cholesterol: 100mg
- Sodium: 180mg
- Total Carbohydrates: 4g
- Dietary Fiber: 0g
- Sugars: 2g
- Protein: 32g

Number of Servings: 4
**Cooking Time: 30 minutes
(plus marinating time)**

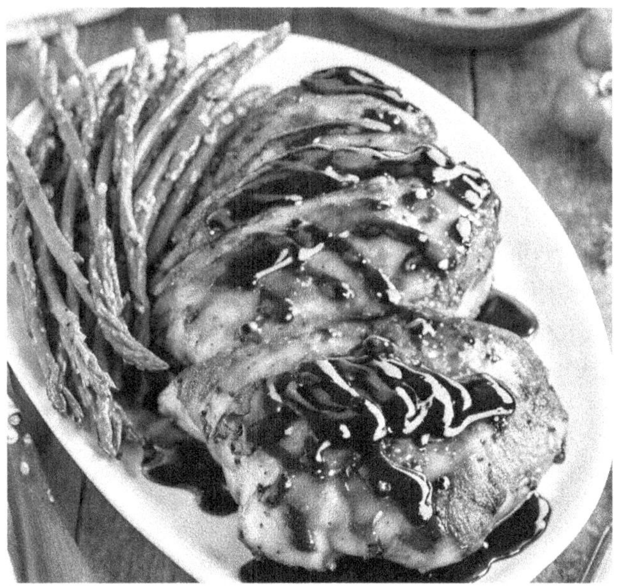

Fish and Seafood Recipes

1. Grilled Salmon with Lemon Butter

Ingredients:

- 4 salmon fillets (6 oz each)
- 1/4 cup butter, melted
- 2 tablespoons lemon juice
- 2 cloves garlic, minced
- 1 tablespoon fresh dill, chopped
- 1 tablespoon olive oil
- 1 lemon, sliced for garnish

Instructions:

1. Preheat your grill to medium-high heat.
2. In a small bowl, combine the melted butter, lemon juice, minced garlic, and chopped dill.
3. Brush the salmon fillets with olive oil.
4. Grill the salmon fillets for 4-5 minutes per side, until the fish is opaque and flakes easily with a fork.
5. During the last minute of grilling, brush the salmon with the lemon butter mixture.
6. Remove from the grill and let rest for a few minutes.
7. Serve garnished with lemon slices.

Nutrition Info Per Serving (1 salmon fillet):

- Calories: 380
- Total Fat: 28g
- Saturated Fat: 12g
- Cholesterol: 100mg
- Sodium: 90mg
- Total Carbohydrates: 2g
- Dietary Fiber: 0g
- Sugars: 0g
- Protein: 30g

Number of Servings: 4
Cooking Time: 10 minutes

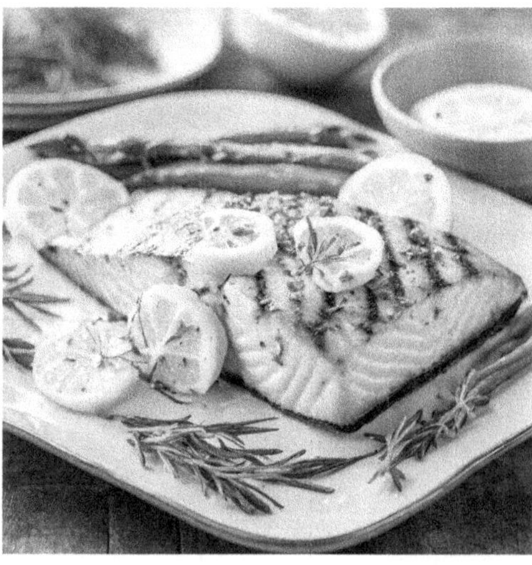

2. Baked Cod with Herb Crust

Ingredients:

- 4 cod fillets (6 oz each)
- 1/4 cup almond flour
- 1/4 cup grated Parmesan cheese
- 2 tablespoons butter, melted
- 1 tablespoon fresh parsley, chopped
- 1 tablespoon fresh thyme, chopped
- 2 cloves garlic, minced
- 1 tablespoon olive oil

Instructions:

1. Preheat your oven to 375°F (190°C).
2. In a small bowl, combine the almond flour, grated Parmesan cheese, melted butter, chopped parsley, chopped thyme, and minced garlic.
3. Brush the cod fillets with olive oil and place them on a baking sheet lined with parchment paper.
4. Press the herb mixture onto the top of each cod fillet.
5. Bake in the preheated oven for 15-20 minutes, until the fish is opaque and flakes easily with a fork.
6. Remove from the oven and let rest for a few minutes before serving.

Nutrition Info Per Serving (1 cod fillet):

- Calories: 280
- Total Fat: 18g
- Saturated Fat: 7g
- Cholesterol: 80mg
- Sodium: 220mg
- Total Carbohydrates: 3g
- Dietary Fiber: 1g
- Sugars: 0g
- Protein: 26g

Number of Servings: 4
Cooking Time: 20 minutes

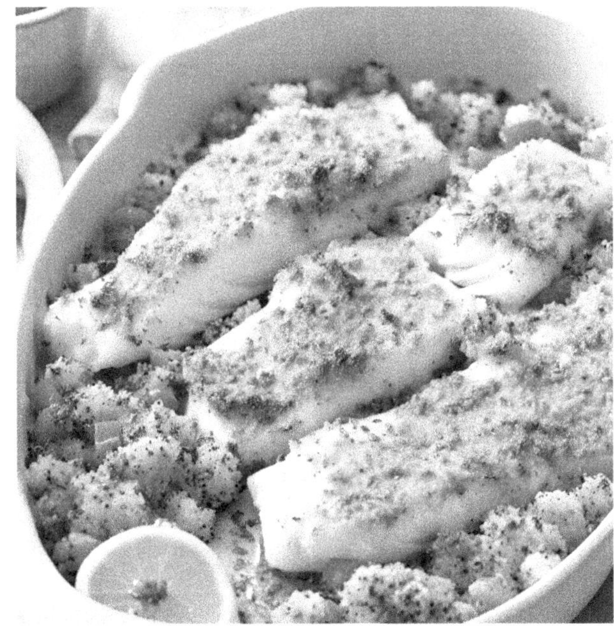

3. Tuna Stuffed Avocado

Ingredients:

- 2 large avocados, halved and pitted
- 1 can (5 oz) tuna, drained
- 1/4 cup mayonnaise (preferably made with avocado oil)
- 1 tablespoon lemon juice
- 1 tablespoon fresh dill, chopped
- 2 green onions, chopped
- 1 clove garlic, minced

Instructions:

1. In a bowl, combine the drained tuna, mayonnaise, lemon juice, chopped dill, chopped green onions, and minced garlic. Mix well.
2. Scoop out a small portion of the avocado flesh to create a larger cavity for the filling.
3. Fill each avocado half with the tuna mixture.
4. Serve immediately.

Nutrition Info Per Serving (1 stuffed avocado half):

- Calories: 320
- Total Fat: 26g
- Saturated Fat: 4g
- Cholesterol: 35mg
- Sodium: 220mg
- Total Carbohydrates: 10g
- Dietary Fiber: 7g
- Sugars: 1g
- Protein: 10g

Number of Servings: 4 Cooking Time: 10 minutes

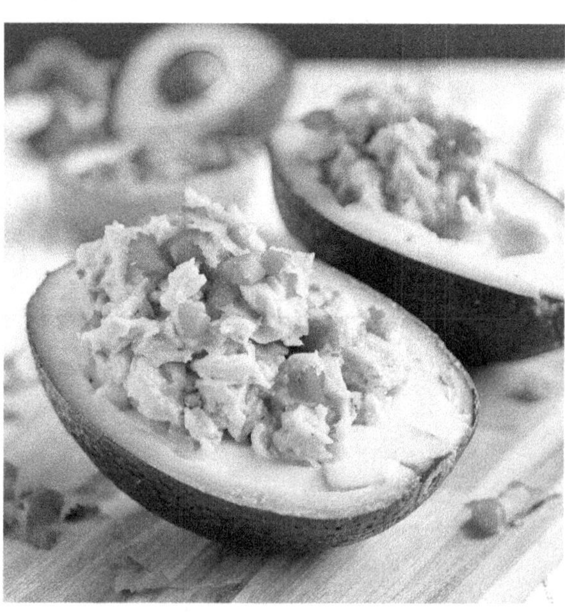

4. Garlic Butter Shrimp Skewers

Ingredients:

- 1 lb large shrimp, peeled and deveined
- 1/4 cup butter, melted
- 3 cloves garlic, minced
- 1 tablespoon lemon juice
- 1 tablespoon fresh parsley, chopped
- 1 tablespoon olive oil

Instructions:

1. Preheat your grill to medium-high heat.
2. In a small bowl, combine the melted butter, minced garlic, lemon juice, and chopped parsley.
3. Thread the shrimp onto skewers.
4. Brush the shrimp with olive oil.
5. Grill the shrimp skewers for 2-3 minutes per side, until the shrimp are pink and opaque.
6. During the last minute of grilling, brush the shrimp with the garlic butter mixture.
7. Remove from the grill and let rest for a few minutes before serving.

Nutrition Info Per Serving (2 skewers):

- Calories: 210
- Total Fat: 16g
- Saturated Fat: 8g
- Cholesterol: 180mg
- Sodium: 220mg
- Total Carbohydrates: 1g
- Dietary Fiber: 0g
- Sugars: 0g
- Protein: 16g

Number of Servings: 4
Cooking Time: 10 minutes

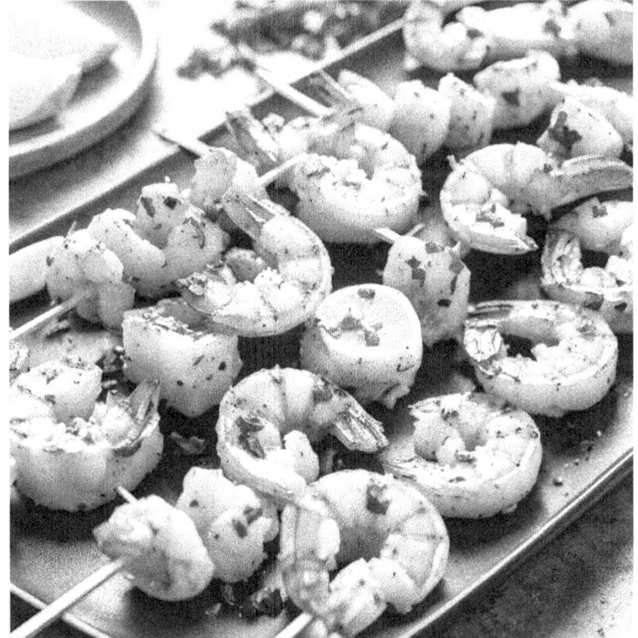

5. Baked Haddock with Creamy Dill Sauce

Ingredients:

- 4 haddock fillets (6 oz each)
- 1/4 cup heavy cream
- 1/4 cup mayonnaise (preferably made with avocado oil)
- 1 tablespoon lemon juice
- 2 tablespoons fresh dill, chopped
- 2 cloves garlic, minced
- 1 tablespoon olive oil

Instructions:

1. Preheat your oven to 375°F (190°C).
2. Place the haddock fillets on a baking sheet lined with parchment paper and brush with olive oil.
3. In a small bowl, mix together the heavy cream, mayonnaise, lemon juice, chopped dill, and minced garlic.
4. Spread the creamy dill mixture evenly over the haddock fillets.
5. Bake in the preheated oven for 15-20 minutes, until the fish is opaque and flakes easily with a fork.
6. Remove from the oven and let rest for a few minutes before serving.

Nutrition Info Per Serving (1 fillet with sauce):

- Calories: 320
- Total Fat: 24g
- Saturated Fat: 10g
- Cholesterol: 110mg
- Sodium: 200mg
- Total Carbohydrates: 2g
- Dietary Fiber: 0g
- Sugars: 0g
- Protein: 24g

Number of Servings: 4
Cooking Time: 20 minutes

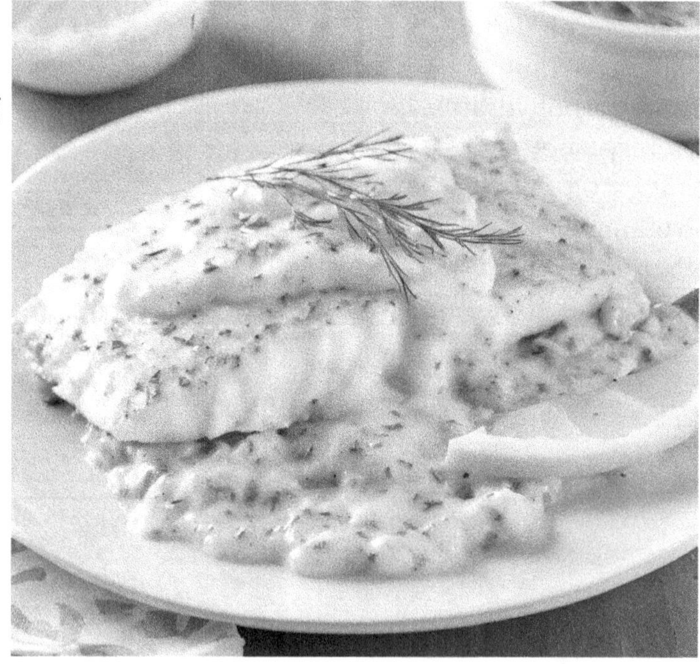

6. Clam Chowder (Low Carb)

Ingredients:

- 2 cups chopped clams (canned or fresh)
- 4 slices bacon, chopped
- 1 small onion, chopped
- 2 cloves garlic, minced
- 1 cup cauliflower florets, finely chopped
- 2 cups heavy cream
- 1 cup chicken broth
- 1/2 cup celery, chopped
- 1 tablespoon fresh thyme, chopped
- 1 tablespoon butter

Instructions:

1. In a large pot, cook the chopped bacon over medium heat until crispy. Remove the bacon and set aside, leaving the rendered fat in the pot.
2. Add the chopped onion, celery, and minced garlic to the pot. Cook until softened, about 5 minutes.
3. Add the finely chopped cauliflower florets and cook for another 3 minutes.
4. Stir in the heavy cream, chicken broth, and chopped thyme. Bring to a simmer.
5. Add the chopped clams and cooked bacon to the pot. Simmer for 10 minutes, stirring occasionally.
6. Stir in the butter until melted and well combined.
7. Serve hot.

Nutrition Info Per Serving (1 cup):

- Calories: 350
- Total Fat: 30g
- Saturated Fat: 15g
- Cholesterol: 110mg
- Sodium: 480mg
- Total Carbohydrates: 6g
- Dietary Fiber: 2g
- Sugars: 2g
- Protein: 14g

Number of Servings: 4

Cooking Time: 20 minutes

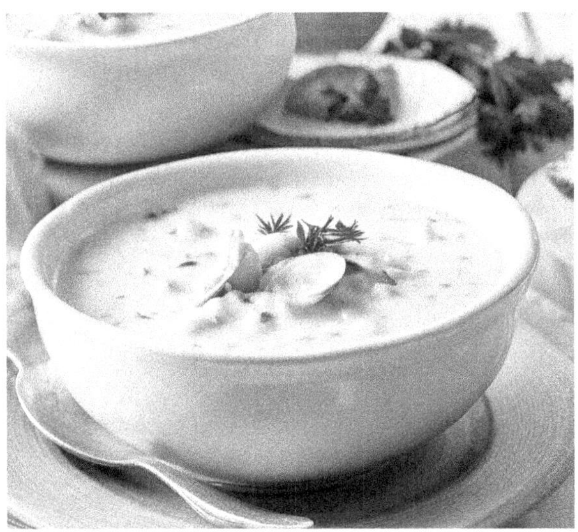

7. Grilled Mackerel with Olive Tapenade

Ingredients:

- 4 mackerel fillets (6 oz each)
- 1/4 cup olive oil
- 2 tablespoons lemon juice
- 1 cup mixed olives, pitted and chopped
- 2 cloves garlic, minced
- 1 tablespoon fresh parsley, chopped
- 1 teaspoon dried oregano

Instructions:

1. Preheat your grill to medium-high heat.
2. In a small bowl, mix together the olive oil, lemon juice, minced garlic, chopped parsley, and dried oregano.
3. Brush the mackerel fillets with the olive oil mixture.
4. Grill the mackerel fillets for 4-5 minutes per side, until the fish is opaque and flakes easily with a fork.
5. In a separate bowl, combine the chopped olives with any remaining olive oil mixture to make the tapenade.
6. Serve the grilled mackerel topped with the olive tapenade.

Nutrition Info Per Serving (1 fillet with tapenade):

- Calories: 380
- Total Fat: 30g
- Saturated Fat: 6g
- Cholesterol: 80mg
- Sodium: 300mg
- Total Carbohydrates: 2g
- Dietary Fiber: 1g
- Sugars: 0g
- Protein: 24g

Number of Servings: 4
Cooking Time: 10 minutes

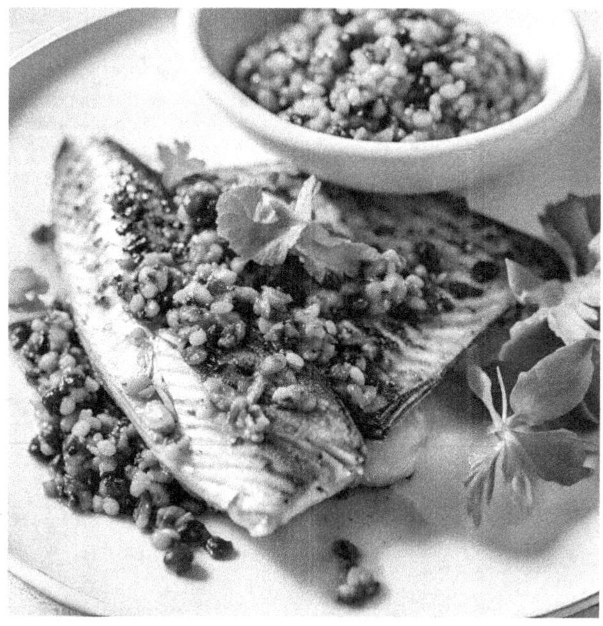

8. Seared Scallops with Bacon

Ingredients:

- 1 lb large sea scallops
- 4 slices bacon, chopped
- 2 tablespoons butter
- 2 cloves garlic, minced
- 1 tablespoon fresh parsley, chopped
- 1 tablespoon lemon juice

Instructions:

1. In a large skillet, cook the chopped bacon over medium heat until crispy. Remove the bacon and set aside, leaving the rendered fat in the skillet.
2. Pat the scallops dry with paper towels and season them with lemon juice.
3. In the same skillet with the bacon fat, add the butter and heat over medium-high heat until melted.
4. Add the scallops to the skillet and sear for 2-3 minutes per side, until a golden crust forms and the scallops are cooked through.
5. Add the minced garlic and chopped parsley to the skillet and cook for an additional 1 minute, stirring frequently.
6. Return the bacon to the skillet and toss to combine.
7. Serve hot.

Nutrition Info Per Serving (4 scallops with bacon):

- Calories: 300
- Total Fat: 22g
- Saturated Fat: 10g
- Cholesterol: 80mg
- Sodium: 340mg
- Total Carbohydrates: 2g
- Dietary Fiber: 0g
- Sugars: 0g
- Protein: 20g

Number of Servings: 4
Cooking Time: 10 minutes

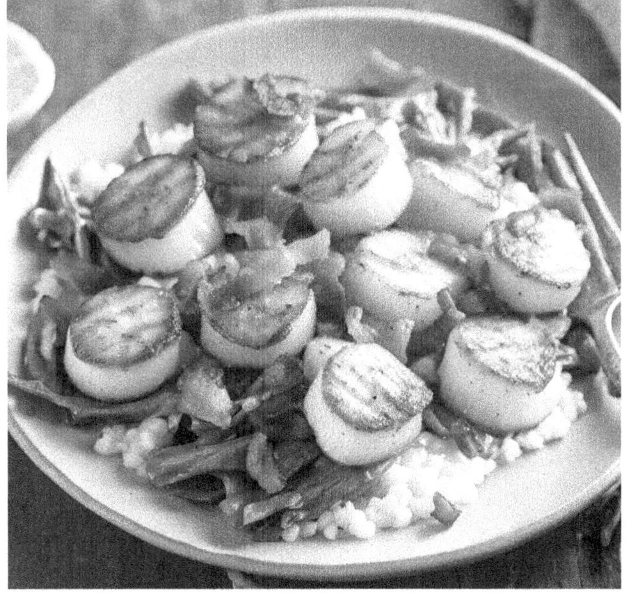

9. Keto Sushi Rolls

Ingredients:
- 4 sheets nori seaweed
- 1 cup cauliflower rice
- 1 tablespoon rice vinegar
- 1 avocado, sliced
- 1 cucumber, julienned
- 4 oz smoked salmon or cooked shrimp
- 1 tablespoon mayonnaise (preferably made with avocado oil)
- 1 tablespoon soy sauce (or coconut aminos)
- 1 tablespoon sesame seeds

Instructions:
1. In a small bowl, mix the cauliflower rice with the rice vinegar.
2. Place a sheet of nori on a bamboo sushi mat.
3. Spread a thin layer of cauliflower rice over the nori, leaving a 1-inch border at the top.
4. Arrange slices of avocado, cucumber, and smoked salmon (or shrimp) along the bottom edge of the nori.
5. Spread a thin layer of mayonnaise over the fillings.
6. Roll the nori tightly around the fillings using the bamboo mat, sealing the edge with a little water.
7. Slice the roll into bite-sized pieces and sprinkle with sesame seeds.
8. Serve with soy sauce (or coconut aminos) on the side.

Nutrition Info Per Serving (1 roll):
- Calories: 200
- Total Fat: 15g
- Saturated Fat: 3g
- Cholesterol: 30mg
- Sodium: 360mg
- Total Carbohydrates: 6g
- Dietary Fiber: 3g
- Sugars: 1g
- Protein: 10g

Number of Servings: 4
Cooking Time: 20 minutes

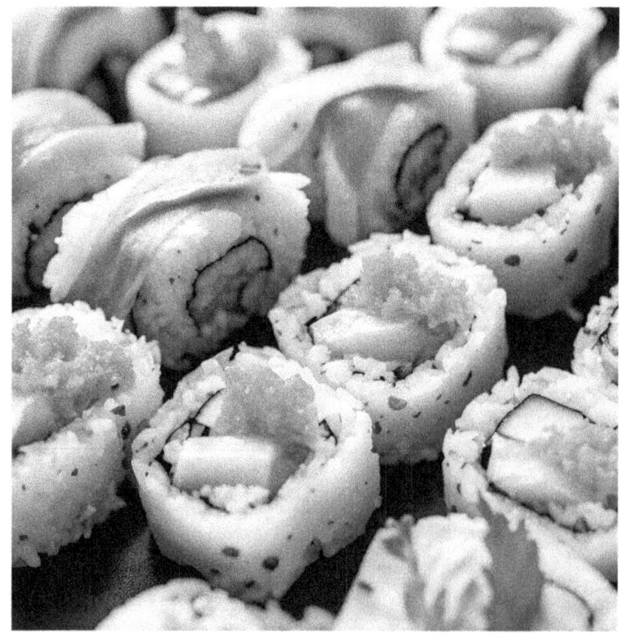

10. Creamy Salmon Florentine

Ingredients:

- 4 salmon fillets (6 oz each)
- 2 tablespoons olive oil
- 2 tablespoons butter
- 2 cloves garlic, minced
- 1 cup heavy cream
- 1/2 cup grated Parmesan cheese
- 1 cup baby spinach
- 1 tablespoon lemon juice

Instructions:

1. Heat the olive oil in a large skillet over medium-high heat.
2. Add the salmon fillets and cook for 4-5 minutes per side, until golden brown and cooked through. Remove from the skillet and set aside.
3. In the same skillet, melt the butter and sauté the minced garlic for 1-2 minutes until fragrant.
4. Stir in the heavy cream and grated Parmesan cheese. Cook for 2-3 minutes until the sauce thickens.
5. Add the baby spinach and cook until wilted, about 1-2 minutes.
6. Stir in the lemon juice.
7. Return the salmon to the skillet and spoon the creamy sauce over the top.
8. Serve hot.

Nutrition Info Per Serving (1 fillet with sauce):

- Calories: 420
- Total Fat: 32g
- Saturated Fat: 15g
- Cholesterol: 120mg
- Sodium: 220mg
- Total Carbohydrates: 3g
- Dietary Fiber: 1g
- Sugars: 1g
- Protein: 30g

Number of Servings: 4
Cooking Time: 15 minutes

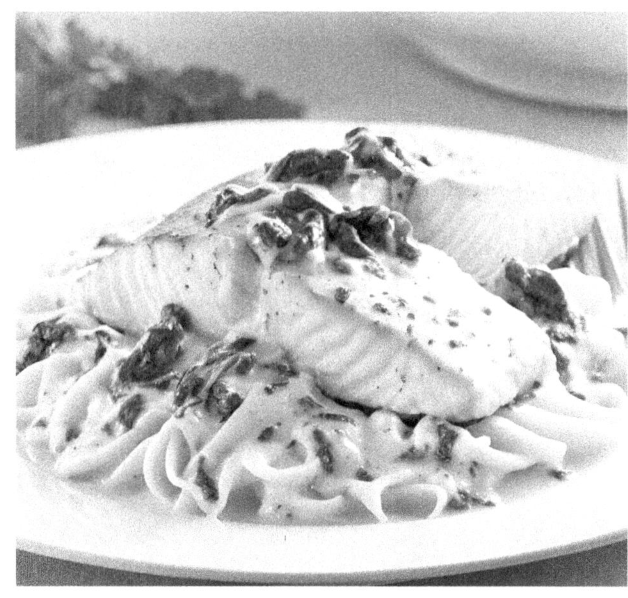

11. Pesto Shrimp with Zoodles

Ingredients:

- 1 lb large shrimp, peeled and deveined
- 4 medium zucchinis, spiralized into zoodles
- 1/4 cup prepared pesto sauce (preferably homemade or low-carb)
- 2 tablespoons olive oil
- 1/4 cup grated Parmesan cheese
- 2 cloves garlic, minced
- 1 tablespoon lemon juice

Instructions:

1. Heat 1 tablespoon of olive oil in a large skillet over medium-high heat.
2. Add the shrimp and cook for 2-3 minutes per side until pink and opaque. Remove from the skillet and set aside.
3. In the same skillet, add the remaining olive oil and minced garlic. Sauté for 1-2 minutes until fragrant.
4. Add the spiralized zucchini and cook for 2-3 minutes until tender.
5. Return the shrimp to the skillet and add the pesto sauce. Toss to coat evenly.
6. Stir in the lemon juice.
7. Sprinkle with grated Parmesan cheese before serving.

Nutrition Info Per Serving (1 bowl):

- Calories: 300
- Total Fat: 20g
- Saturated Fat: 5g
- Cholesterol: 180mg
- Sodium: 350mg
- Total Carbohydrates: 6g
- Dietary Fiber: 2g
- Sugars: 3g
- Protein: 25g

Number of Servings: 4
Cooking Time: 15 minutes

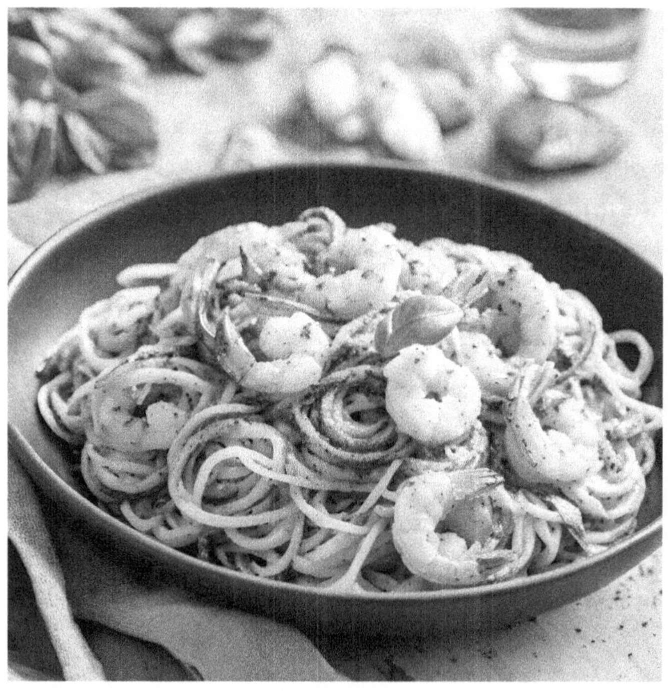

12. Smoked Trout with Cream Cheese Spread

Ingredients:

- 4 smoked trout fillets
- 1 cup cream cheese, softened
- 2 tablespoons heavy cream
- 2 tablespoons fresh dill, chopped
- 1 tablespoon lemon juice
- 1 clove garlic, minced

Instructions:

1. In a mixing bowl, combine the softened cream cheese, heavy cream, chopped dill, lemon juice, and minced garlic. Mix until smooth and creamy.
2. Spread the cream cheese mixture evenly over the smoked trout fillets.
3. Garnish with additional fresh dill if desired.
4. Serve immediately.

Nutrition Info Per Serving (1 fillet with spread):

- Calories: 320
- Total Fat: 26g
- Saturated Fat: 12g
- Cholesterol: 100mg
- Sodium: 240mg
- Total Carbohydrates: 3g
- Dietary Fiber: 0g
- Sugars: 1g
- Protein: 20g

Number of Servings: 4

Cooking Time: 10 minutes

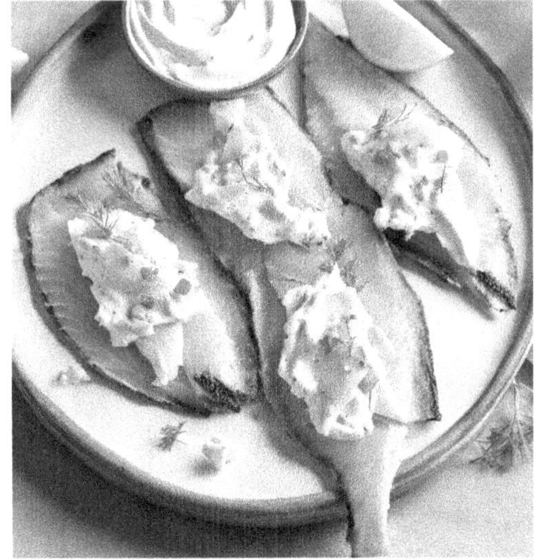

13. Anchovy and Garlic Stuffed Olives
Ingredients:

- 1 jar (8 oz) large green olives, pitted
- 1 can (2 oz) anchovy fillets, drained and finely chopped
- 2 cloves garlic, minced
- 1 tablespoon olive oil

Instructions:

1. In a small bowl, combine the finely chopped anchovy fillets, minced garlic, and olive oil. Mix well.
2. Using a small spoon or piping bag, stuff each olive with the anchovy and garlic mixture.
3. Serve immediately or refrigerate until ready to serve.

Nutrition Info Per Serving (10 olives):

- Calories: 90
- Total Fat: 8g
- Saturated Fat: 1g
- Cholesterol: 10mg
- Sodium: 480mg
- Total Carbohydrates: 1g
- Dietary Fiber: 0g
- Sugars: 0g
- Protein: 3g

Number of Servings: 4
Cooking Time: 10 minutes

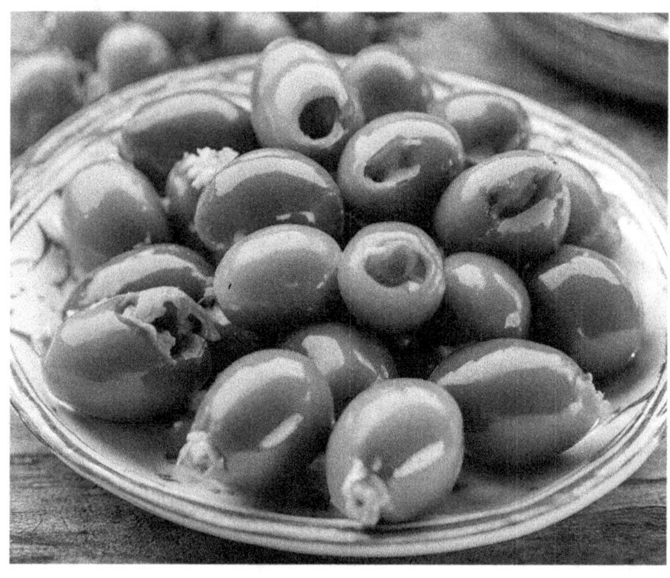

14. Mussels in Garlic Butter Sauce

Ingredients:

- 2 lbs fresh mussels, scrubbed and debearded
- 1/4 cup butter
- 4 cloves garlic, minced
- 1/2 cup dry white wine
- 1/4 cup heavy cream
- 2 tablespoons fresh parsley, chopped
- 1 tablespoon lemon juice

Instructions:

1. In a large pot, melt the butter over medium heat.
2. Add the minced garlic and sauté for 1-2 minutes until fragrant.
3. Pour in the white wine and bring to a simmer.
4. Add the mussels to the pot, cover, and cook for 5-7 minutes until the mussels open.
5. Remove the mussels from the pot with a slotted spoon and set aside.
6. Stir the heavy cream and lemon juice into the pot and simmer for an additional 2-3 minutes.
7. Return the mussels to the pot and toss to coat with the sauce.
8. Garnish with chopped parsley before serving.

Nutrition Info Per Serving (1 cup):

- Calories: 280
- Total Fat: 20g
- Saturated Fat: 10g
- Cholesterol: 85mg
- Sodium: 500mg
- Total Carbohydrates: 3g
- Dietary Fiber: 0g
- Sugars: 1g
- Protein: 20g

Number of Servings: 4
Cooking Time: 15 minutes

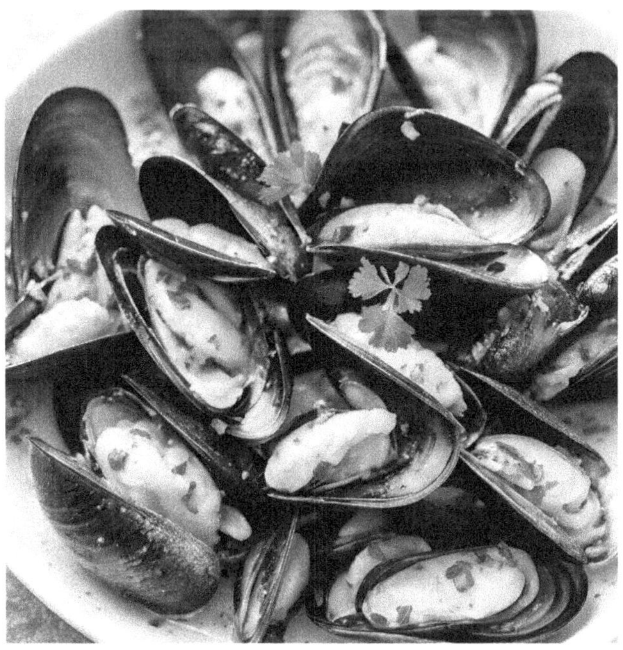

15. Fish Piccata

Ingredients:

- 4 white fish fillets (such as cod or tilapia)
- 1/4 cup almond flour
- 2 tablespoons olive oil
- 1/4 cup butter
- 3 cloves garlic, minced
- 1/2 cup chicken broth
- 1/4 cup lemon juice
- 2 tablespoons capers, drained
- 2 tablespoons fresh parsley, chopped

Instructions:

1. Lightly coat the fish fillets with almond flour.
2. Heat the olive oil in a large skillet over medium-high heat.
3. Add the fish fillets and cook for 3-4 minutes per side until golden brown and cooked through. Remove from the skillet and set aside.
4. In the same skillet, melt the butter and sauté the minced garlic for 1-2 minutes until fragrant.
5. Pour in the chicken broth and lemon juice, stirring to deglaze the pan.
6. Stir in the capers and cook for another 2-3 minutes until the sauce thickens slightly.
7. Return the fish fillets to the skillet and spoon the sauce over them.
8. Garnish with chopped parsley before serving.

Nutrition Info Per Serving (1 fillet with sauce):

- Calories: 350
- Total Fat: 28g
- Saturated Fat: 10g
- Cholesterol: 85mg
- Sodium: 340mg
- Total Carbohydrates: 4g
- Dietary Fiber: 1g
- Sugars: 1g
- Protein: 20g

Number of Servings: 4
Cooking Time: 20 minutes

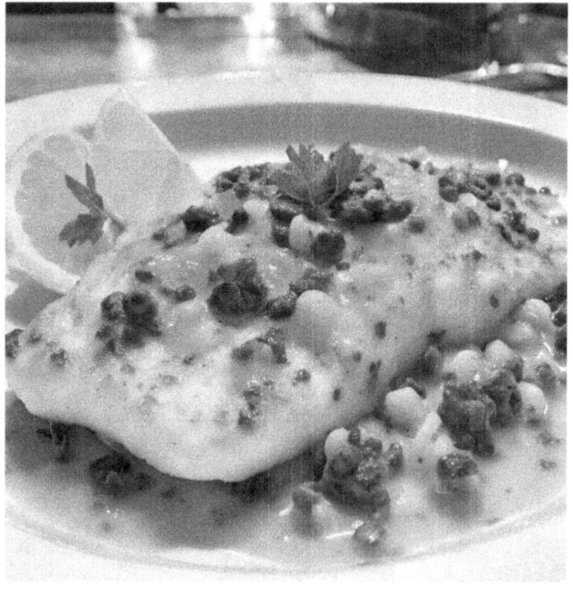

16. Salmon Patties with Dill Sauce

Ingredients:

- 1 lb canned salmon, drained and flaked
- 1/4 cup almond flour
- 2 large eggs, beaten
- 1/4 cup green onions, chopped
- 2 tablespoons mayonnaise (preferably made with avocado oil)
- 2 tablespoons fresh dill, chopped
- 2 tablespoons butter

For the Dill Sauce:

- 1/2 cup sour cream
- 2 tablespoons mayonnaise (preferably made with avocado oil)
- 1 tablespoon lemon juice
- 1 tablespoon fresh dill, chopped
- 1 clove garlic, minced

Instructions:

1. In a large mixing bowl, combine the flaked salmon, almond flour, beaten eggs, chopped green onions, mayonnaise, and fresh dill. Mix well to form a cohesive mixture.
2. Shape the mixture into 8 patties.
3. Heat the butter in a large skillet over medium-high heat.
4. Add the salmon patties to the skillet and cook for 3-4 minutes per side, until golden brown and cooked through. Remove from the skillet and set aside.
5. While the patties are cooking, prepare the dill sauce. In a small bowl, combine the sour cream, mayonnaise, lemon juice, chopped dill, and minced garlic. Mix well.
6. Serve the salmon patties hot, topped with the dill sauce.

Nutrition Info Per Serving (2 patties with sauce):

- Calories: 350
- Total Fat: 28g
- Saturated Fat: 10g
- Cholesterol: 110mg
- Sodium: 340mg
- Total Carbohydrates: 4g
- Dietary Fiber: 1g
- Sugars: 1g
- Protein: 20g

Number of Servings: 4

Cooking Time: 20 minutes

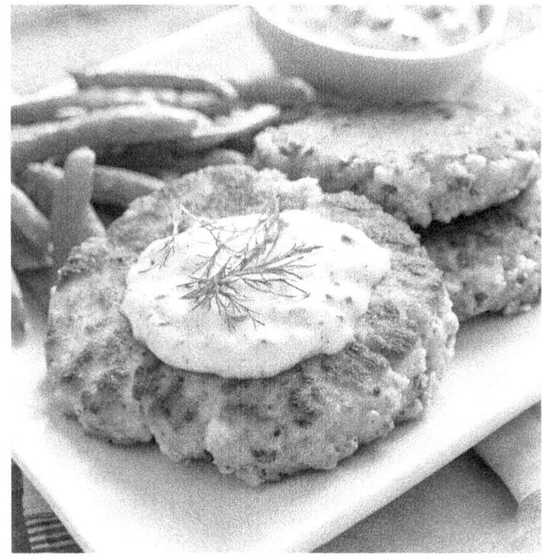

17. Keto Paella

Ingredients:

- 1 lb shrimp, peeled and deveined
- 1 lb mussels, cleaned
- 1 lb chicken thighs, cut into bite-sized pieces
- 1 cup cauliflower rice
- 1 red bell pepper, chopped
- 1 small onion, chopped
- 3 cloves garlic, minced
- 1/4 cup olive oil
- 1/2 cup chicken broth
- 1/4 cup heavy cream
- 1/2 teaspoon saffron threads
- 1 teaspoon smoked paprika
- 1 teaspoon dried oregano
- 1/4 cup fresh parsley, chopped

Instructions:

1. In a large skillet, heat the olive oil over medium-high heat.
2. Add the chicken pieces and cook until browned, about 5-7 minutes. Remove from the skillet and set aside.
3. In the same skillet, add the chopped onion, red bell pepper, and minced garlic. Sauté for 3-4 minutes until softened.
4. Stir in the cauliflower rice, smoked paprika, dried oregano, and saffron threads. Cook for 2-3 minutes.
5. Add the chicken broth and heavy cream, stirring to combine.
6. Return the chicken to the skillet, along with the shrimp and mussels. Cover and cook for 5-7 minutes until the shrimp are pink and the mussels have opened.
7. Remove from heat and garnish with fresh parsley before serving.

Nutrition Info Per Serving (1 cup):

- Calories: 350
- Total Fat: 24g
- Saturated Fat: 7g
- Cholesterol: 220mg
- Sodium: 500mg
- Total Carbohydrates: 6g
- Dietary Fiber: 2g
- Sugars: 2g
- Protein: 28g

Number of Servings: 4

Cooking Time: 30 minutes

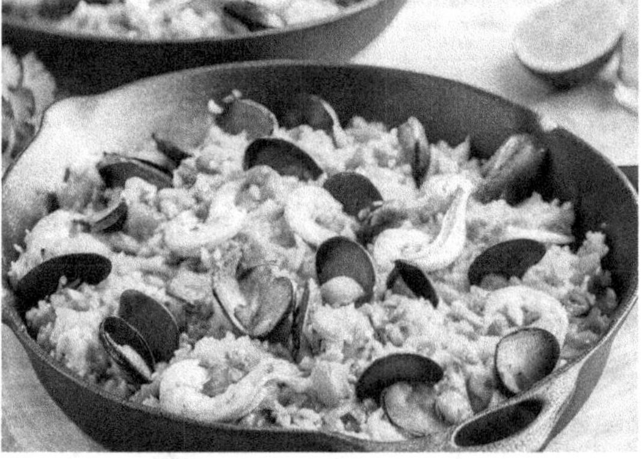

18. Baked Lemon-Garlic Tilapia

Ingredients:

- 4 tilapia fillets (6 oz each)
- 1/4 cup butter, melted
- 2 tablespoons lemon juice
- 3 cloves garlic, minced
- 1 tablespoon fresh parsley, chopped
- 1 teaspoon dried oregano

Instructions:

1. Preheat your oven to 375°F (190°C).
2. In a small bowl, combine the melted butter, lemon juice, minced garlic, chopped parsley, and dried oregano.
3. Place the tilapia fillets on a baking sheet lined with parchment paper.
4. Pour the lemon-garlic butter mixture over the tilapia fillets.
5. Bake in the preheated oven for 15-20 minutes until the fish is opaque and flakes easily with a fork.
6. Remove from the oven and let rest for a few minutes before serving.

Nutrition Info Per Serving (1 fillet):

- Calories: 280
- Total Fat: 20g
- Saturated Fat: 10g
- Cholesterol: 90mg
- Sodium: 150mg
- Total Carbohydrates: 2g
- Dietary Fiber: 0g
- Sugars: 0g
- Protein: 22g

Number of Servings: 4
Cooking Time: 20 minutes

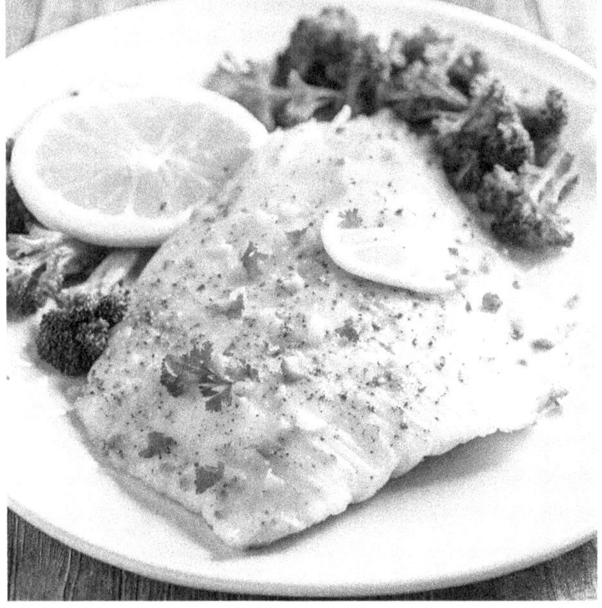

19. Parmesan Crusted Flounder

Ingredients:

- 4 flounder fillets (6 oz each)
- 1/2 cup grated Parmesan cheese
- 1/4 cup almond flour
- 2 tablespoons butter, melted
- 2 cloves garlic, minced
- 1 tablespoon fresh parsley, chopped
- 1 tablespoon olive oil

Instructions:

1. Preheat your oven to 400°F (200°C).
2. In a small bowl, combine the grated Parmesan cheese, almond flour, melted butter, minced garlic, and chopped parsley.
3. Brush the flounder fillets with olive oil and place them on a baking sheet lined with parchment paper.
4. Press the Parmesan mixture onto the top of each flounder fillet.
5. Bake in the preheated oven for 12-15 minutes until the crust is golden and the fish is cooked through.
6. Remove from the oven and let rest for a few minutes before serving.

Nutrition Info Per Serving (1 fillet):

- Calories: 320
- Total Fat: 22g
- Saturated Fat: 9g
- Cholesterol: 85mg
- Sodium: 220mg
- Total Carbohydrates: 2g
- Dietary Fiber: 1g
- Sugars: 0g
- Protein: 26g

Number of Servings: 4
Cooking Time: 15 minutes

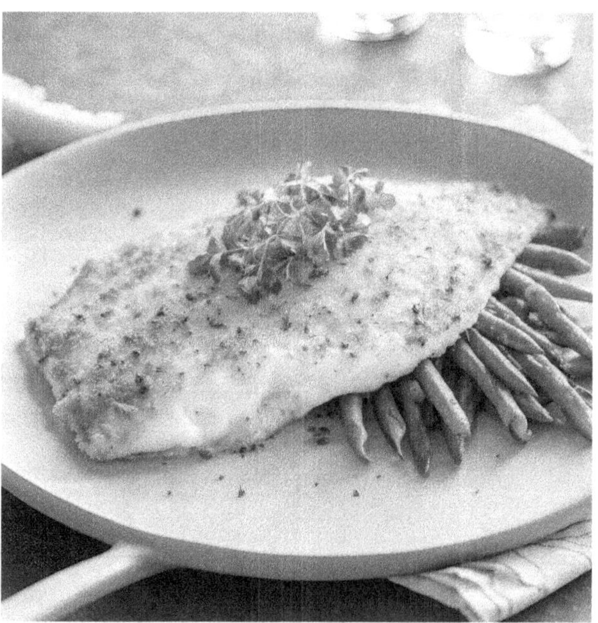

20. Halibut Steak with Capers

Ingredients:

- 4 halibut steaks (6 oz each)
- 1/4 cup olive oil
- 2 tablespoons butter
- 3 cloves garlic, minced
- 1/4 cup lemon juice
- 2 tablespoons capers, drained
- 1 tablespoon fresh parsley, chopped

Instructions:

1. Heat the olive oil in a large skillet over medium-high heat.
2. Add the halibut steaks and cook for 4-5 minutes per side until golden brown and cooked through. Remove from the skillet and set aside.
3. In the same skillet, melt the butter and sauté the minced garlic for 1-2 minutes until fragrant.
4. Stir in the lemon juice and capers, cooking for an additional 2 minutes.
5. Return the halibut steaks to the skillet and spoon the sauce over them.
6. Garnish with chopped parsley before serving.

Nutrition Info Per Serving (1 steak with sauce):

- Calories: 380
- Total Fat: 28g
- Saturated Fat: 10g
- Cholesterol: 80mg
- Sodium: 300mg
- Total Carbohydrates: 2g
- Dietary Fiber: 0g
- Sugars: 0g
- Protein: 28g

Number of Servings: 4
Cooking Time: 15 minutes

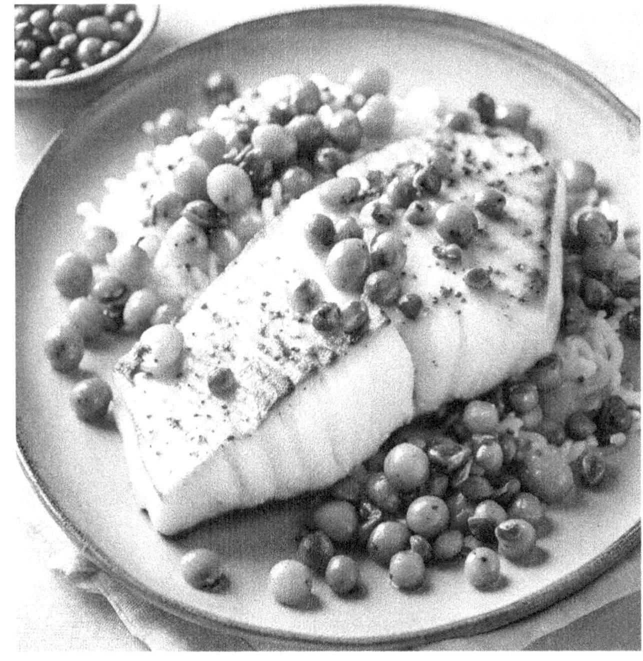

21. Keto Fish and Chips

Ingredients:

For the Fish:

- 4 white fish fillets (such as cod or haddock)
- 1 cup almond flour
- 1/4 cup grated Parmesan cheese
- 2 large eggs, beaten
- 1/4 cup heavy cream
- 1/4 cup coconut oil (or other high-heat oil) for frying

For the Chips:

- 2 medium turnips, peeled and cut into fries
- 2 tablespoons olive oil
- 1 teaspoon paprika

Instructions:

For the Fish:

1. In a shallow dish, combine the almond flour and grated Parmesan cheese.
2. In another bowl, whisk together the eggs and heavy cream.
3. Dip each fish fillet into the egg mixture, then coat with the almond flour mixture.
4. Heat the coconut oil in a large skillet over medium-high heat.
5. Fry the fish fillets for 4-5 minutes per side until golden brown and cooked through. Remove from the skillet and let rest on a paper towel-lined plate.

For the Chips:

1. Preheat your oven to 425°F (220°C).
2. In a large bowl, toss the turnip fries with olive oil and paprika.
3. Spread the turnip fries in a single layer on a baking sheet lined with parchment paper.
4. Bake in the preheated oven for 20-25 minutes, turning halfway through, until crispy and golden.
5. Serve the fish with the turnip chips.

Nutrition Info Per Serving (1 fillet with chips):

- Calories: 450
- Total Fat: 32g
- Saturated Fat: 12g
- Cholesterol: 110mg
- Sodium: 250mg
- Total Carbohydrates: 8g
- Dietary Fiber: 3g
- Sugars: 2g
- Protein: 30g

Number of Servings: 4

Cooking Time: 30 minutes

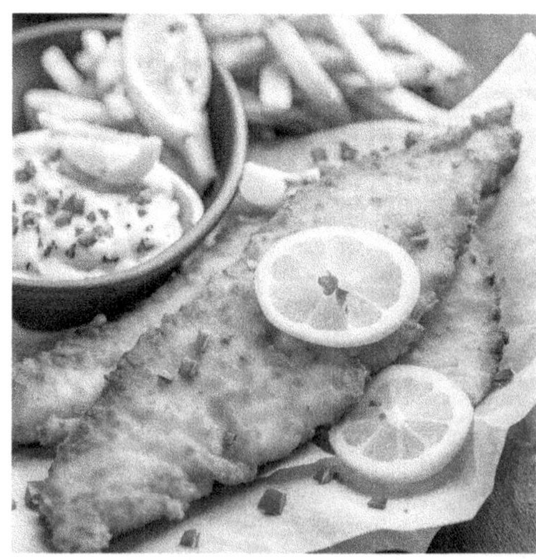

Vegetables

1. Creamed Spinach

Ingredients:

- 2 lbs fresh spinach, washed and trimmed
- 1/4 cup butter
- 1 cup heavy cream
- 1/2 cup grated Parmesan cheese
- 3 cloves garlic, minced
- 1/4 teaspoon ground nutmeg

Instructions:

1. In a large pot, bring water to a boil and add the spinach. Cook for 2-3 minutes until wilted. Drain and squeeze out excess water. Chop the spinach and set aside.
2. In a large skillet, melt the butter over medium heat.
3. Add the minced garlic and sauté for 1-2 minutes until fragrant.
4. Stir in the heavy cream and bring to a simmer.
5. Add the chopped spinach, grated Parmesan cheese, and ground nutmeg. Stir well to combine.
6. Cook for an additional 5 minutes, stirring occasionally, until the mixture thickens.
7. Serve hot.

Nutrition Info Per Serving (1/2 cup):

- Calories: 180
- Total Fat: 16g
- Saturated Fat: 10g
- Cholesterol: 50mg
- Sodium: 180mg
- Total Carbohydrates: 4g
- Dietary Fiber: 2g
- Sugars: 1g
- Protein: 6g

Number of Servings: 6
Cooking Time: 15 minutes

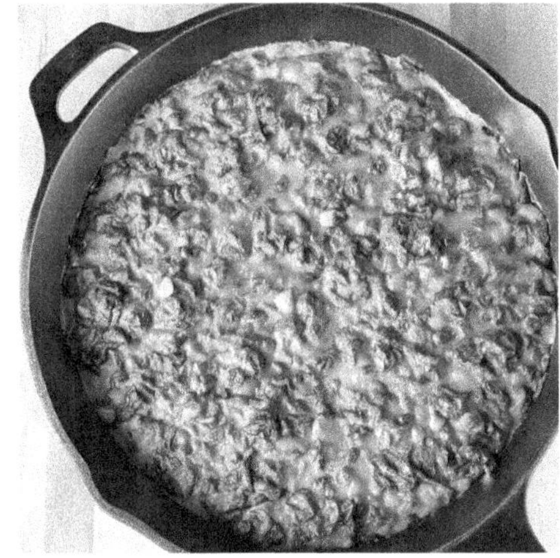

2. Cauliflower Rice

Ingredients:

- 1 large head cauliflower, cut into florets
- 2 tablespoons butter
- 1 tablespoon olive oil
- 2 cloves garlic, minced
- 1/4 cup grated Parmesan cheese

Instructions:

1. Place the cauliflower florets in a food processor and pulse until they resemble rice grains.
2. Heat the butter and olive oil in a large skillet over medium heat.
3. Add the minced garlic and sauté for 1-2 minutes until fragrant.
4. Add the cauliflower rice to the skillet and cook for 5-7 minutes, stirring occasionally, until tender.
5. Stir in the grated Parmesan cheese and cook for an additional 2 minutes.
6. Serve hot.

Nutrition Info Per Serving (1 cup):

- Calories: 120
- Total Fat: 10g
- Saturated Fat: 5g
- Cholesterol: 20mg
- Sodium: 160mg
- Total Carbohydrates: 5g
- Dietary Fiber: 2g
- Sugars: 2g
- Protein: 4g

Number of Servings: 4
Cooking Time: 10 minutes

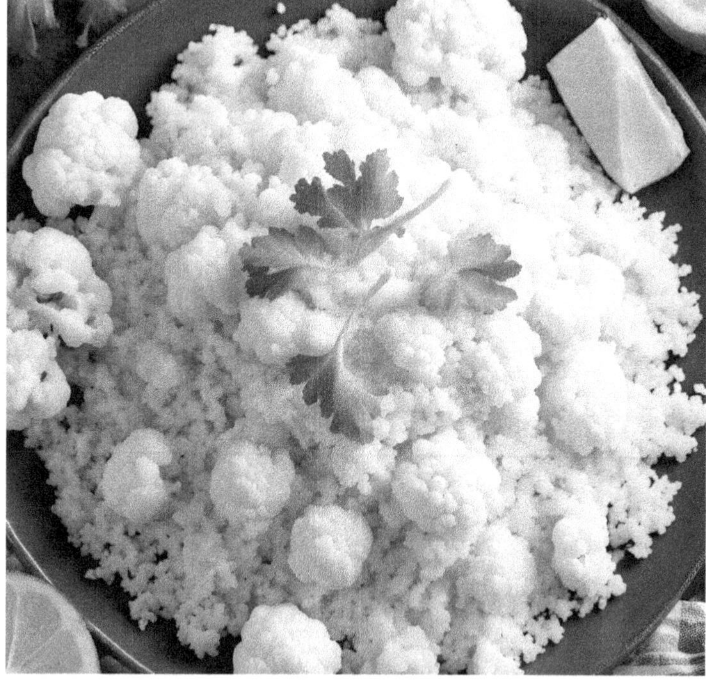

3. Zucchini Noodles with Pesto

Ingredients:

- 4 medium zucchinis, spiralized into noodles
- 1/2 cup prepared pesto sauce (preferably homemade or low-carb)
- 2 tablespoons olive oil
- 1/4 cup grated Parmesan cheese
- 2 cloves garlic, minced

Instructions:

1. Heat the olive oil in a large skillet over medium-high heat.
2. Add the minced garlic and sauté for 1-2 minutes until fragrant.
3. Add the zucchini noodles to the skillet and cook for 2-3 minutes until tender.
4. Remove from heat and toss with the prepared pesto sauce.
5. Sprinkle with grated Parmesan cheese before serving.

Nutrition Info Per Serving (1 cup):

- Calories: 220
- Total Fat: 18g
- Saturated Fat: 4g
- Cholesterol: 10mg
- Sodium: 140mg
- Total Carbohydrates: 6g
- Dietary Fiber: 2g
- Sugars: 3g
- Protein: 6g

Number of Servings: 4 Cooking Time: 10 minutes

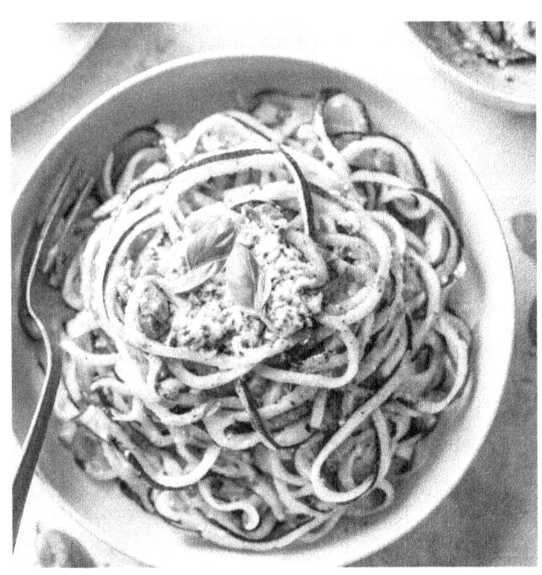

4. Eggplant Lasagna

Ingredients:

- 2 large eggplants, sliced lengthwise into 1/4-inch thick slices
- 1 lb ground beef
- 1 cup marinara sauce (no added sugar)
- 1 cup ricotta cheese
- 1 cup shredded mozzarella cheese
- 1/2 cup grated Parmesan cheese
- 2 cloves garlic, minced
- 2 tablespoons olive oil
- 1 tablespoon dried oregano

Instructions:

1. Preheat your oven to 375°F (190°C).
2. Place the eggplant slices on a baking sheet and brush with olive oil. Bake for 15 minutes until tender.
3. While the eggplant is baking, cook the ground beef in a large skillet over medium-high heat until browned, about 7-10 minutes. Drain any excess fat.
4. Add the minced garlic and marinara sauce to the skillet with the beef. Cook for 5 minutes until heated through.
5. In a 9x13-inch baking dish, spread a layer of the meat sauce on the bottom.
6. Place a layer of eggplant slices over the meat sauce.
7. Spread a layer of ricotta cheese over the eggplant slices, followed by a layer of shredded mozzarella.
8. Repeat the layers until all ingredients are used, finishing with a layer of shredded mozzarella and grated Parmesan on top.
9. Sprinkle the dried oregano over the top.
10. Bake in the preheated oven for 25-30 minutes until the cheese is melted and bubbly.
11. Let the lasagna rest for 10 minutes before slicing and serving.

Nutrition Info Per Serving (1 slice):

- Calories: 400
- Total Fat: 28g
- Saturated Fat: 12g
- Cholesterol: 80mg
- Sodium: 380mg
- Total Carbohydrates: 10g
- Dietary Fiber: 4g
- Sugars: 5g
- Protein: 20g

Number of Servings: 6

Cooking Time: 45 minutes

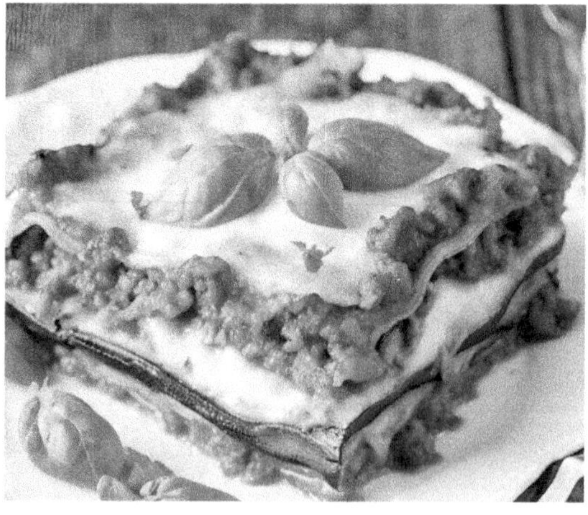

5. Cucumber Salad with Sour Cream and Dill
Ingredients:

- 2 large cucumbers, thinly sliced
- 1 cup sour cream
- 2 tablespoons fresh dill, chopped
- 1 tablespoon apple cider vinegar
- 1 clove garlic, minced

Instructions:

1. In a large bowl, combine the sour cream, chopped dill, apple cider vinegar, and minced garlic.
2. Add the cucumber slices and toss to coat evenly.
3. Chill in the refrigerator for at least 30 minutes before serving.

Nutrition Info Per Serving (1 cup):

- Calories: 90
- Total Fat: 7g
- Saturated Fat: 4g
- Cholesterol: 20mg
- Sodium: 20mg
- Total Carbohydrates: 5g
- Dietary Fiber: 1g
- Sugars: 3g
- Protein: 2g

Number of Servings: 4
Cooking Time: 10 minutes (plus chilling time)

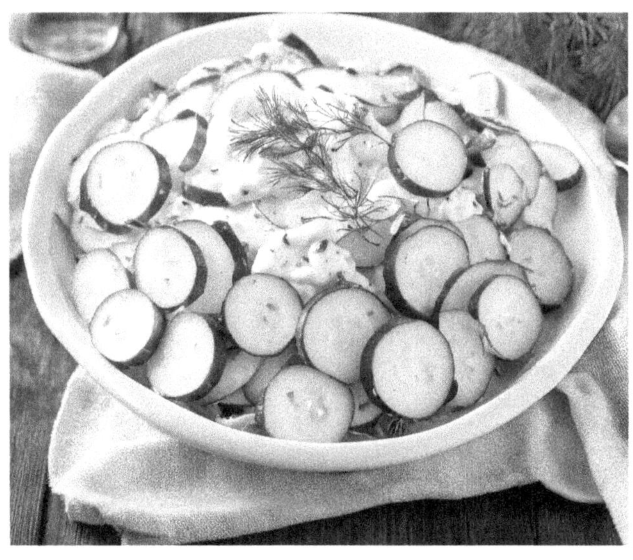

6. Roasted Cauliflower with Turmeric and Cumin

Ingredients:

- 1 large head cauliflower, cut into florets
- 1/4 cup olive oil
- 1 teaspoon ground turmeric
- 1 teaspoon ground cumin
- 2 cloves garlic, minced

Instructions:

1. Preheat your oven to 400°F (200°C).
2. In a large bowl, combine the olive oil, ground turmeric, ground cumin, and minced garlic.
3. Add the cauliflower florets and toss to coat evenly.
4. Spread the cauliflower on a baking sheet lined with parchment paper.
5. Roast in the preheated oven for 25-30 minutes, until golden brown and tender.
6. Serve hot.

Nutrition Info Per Serving (1 cup):

- Calories: 130
- Total Fat: 11g
- Saturated Fat: 1.5g
- Cholesterol: 0mg
- Sodium: 20mg
- Total Carbohydrates: 8g
- Dietary Fiber: 3g
- Sugars: 2g
- Protein: 3g

Number of Servings: 4 Cooking Time: 30 minutes

7. Spaghetti Squash Carbonara

Ingredients:

- 1 large spaghetti squash
- 4 slices bacon, chopped
- 1/2 cup heavy cream
- 1/2 cup grated Parmesan cheese
- 2 large eggs
- 2 cloves garlic, minced
- 1 tablespoon olive oil

Instructions:

1. Preheat your oven to 375°F (190°C).
2. Cut the spaghetti squash in half lengthwise and remove the seeds.
3. Brush the inside of the squash with olive oil and place it cut-side down on a baking sheet.
4. Roast in the preheated oven for 40-45 minutes, until the squash is tender.
5. While the squash is roasting, cook the bacon in a large skillet over medium heat until crispy. Remove from the skillet and set aside, leaving the bacon fat in the skillet.
6. In the same skillet, sauté the minced garlic for 1-2 minutes until fragrant.
7. In a small bowl, whisk together the heavy cream, grated Parmesan cheese, and eggs.
8. Once the squash is done, use a fork to scrape out the strands into a large bowl.
9. Add the bacon, garlic, and cream mixture to the bowl and toss to combine. The heat from the squash will cook the eggs and create a creamy sauce.
10. Serve hot.

Nutrition Info Per Serving (1 cup):

- Calories: 280
- Total Fat: 22g
- Saturated Fat: 10g
- Cholesterol: 130mg
- Sodium: 280mg
- Total Carbohydrates: 10g
- Dietary Fiber: 3g
- Sugars: 3g
- Protein: 10g

Number of Servings: 4

Cooking Time: 45 minutes

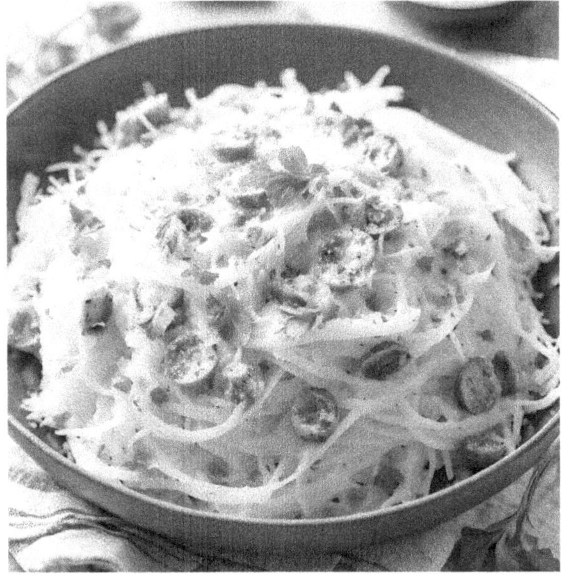

8. Garlic Parmesan Green Beans

Ingredients:

- 1 lb fresh green beans, trimmed
- 2 tablespoons butter
- 2 tablespoons olive oil
- 3 cloves garlic, minced
- 1/4 cup grated Parmesan cheese

Instructions:

1. Bring a large pot of water to a boil. Add the green beans and cook for 3-4 minutes until tender-crisp. Drain and set aside.
2. In a large skillet, melt the butter and olive oil over medium heat.
3. Add the minced garlic and sauté for 1-2 minutes until fragrant.
4. Add the green beans to the skillet and toss to coat with the garlic butter.
5. Sprinkle with grated Parmesan cheese and cook for an additional 2-3 minutes until the cheese is melted.
6. Serve hot.

Nutrition Info Per Serving (1 cup):

- Calories: 160
- Total Fat: 13g
- Saturated Fat: 6g
- Cholesterol: 20mg
- Sodium: 120mg
- Total Carbohydrates: 7g
- Dietary Fiber: 3g
- Sugars: 2g
- Protein: 4g

Number of Servings: 4
Cooking Time: 10 minutes

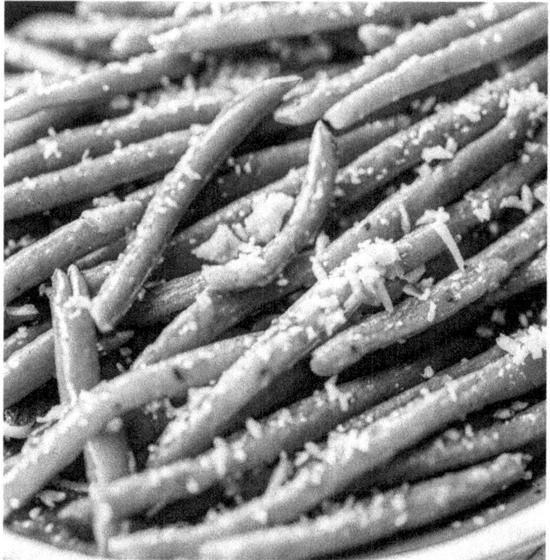

9. Zucchini and Walnut Salad

Ingredients:

- 2 large zucchinis, thinly sliced
- 1/2 cup walnuts, chopped
- 1/4 cup olive oil
- 2 tablespoons lemon juice
- 1 tablespoon fresh parsley, chopped
- 1 clove garlic, minced

Instructions:

1. In a large bowl, combine the olive oil, lemon juice, minced garlic, and chopped parsley.
2. Add the sliced zucchinis and chopped walnuts to the bowl and toss to coat evenly.
3. Chill in the refrigerator for at least 30 minutes before serving.

Nutrition Info Per Serving (1 cup):

- Calories: 200
- Total Fat: 18g
- Saturated Fat: 2g
- Cholesterol: 0mg
- Sodium: 10mg
- Total Carbohydrates: 6g
- Dietary Fiber: 2g
- Sugars: 3g
- Protein: 4g

Number of Servings: 4

Cooking Time: 10 minutes (plus chilling time)

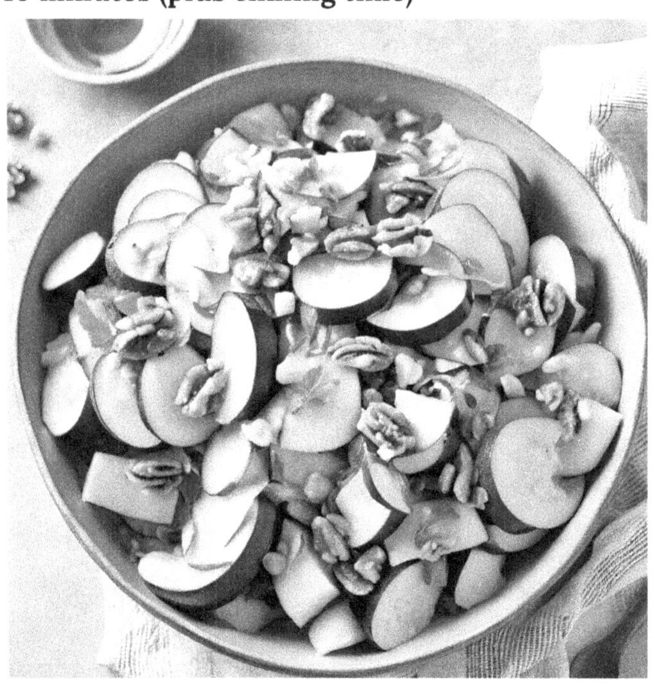

10. Keto Vegetable Stir Fry

Ingredients:

- 1 cup broccoli florets
- 1 cup bell pepper, sliced
- 1 cup snow peas
- 1 cup mushrooms, sliced
- 1/4 cup soy sauce (or coconut aminos)
- 2 tablespoons olive oil
- 2 cloves garlic, minced
- 1 tablespoon ginger, grated
- 1 tablespoon sesame oil

Instructions:

1. Heat the olive oil in a large skillet or wok over medium-high heat.
2. Add the minced garlic and grated ginger, and sauté for 1-2 minutes until fragrant.
3. Add the broccoli, bell pepper, snow peas, and mushrooms to the skillet. Stir-fry for 5-7 minutes until the vegetables are tender-crisp.
4. Stir in the soy sauce (or coconut aminos) and sesame oil. Cook for an additional 2-3 minutes.
5. Serve hot.

Nutrition Info Per Serving (1 cup):

- Calories: 120
- Total Fat: 9g
- Saturated Fat: 1.5g
- Cholesterol: 0mg
- Sodium: 450mg
- Total Carbohydrates: 9g
- Dietary Fiber: 3g
- Sugars: 4g
- Protein: 3g

Number of Servings: 4
Cooking Time: 15 minutes

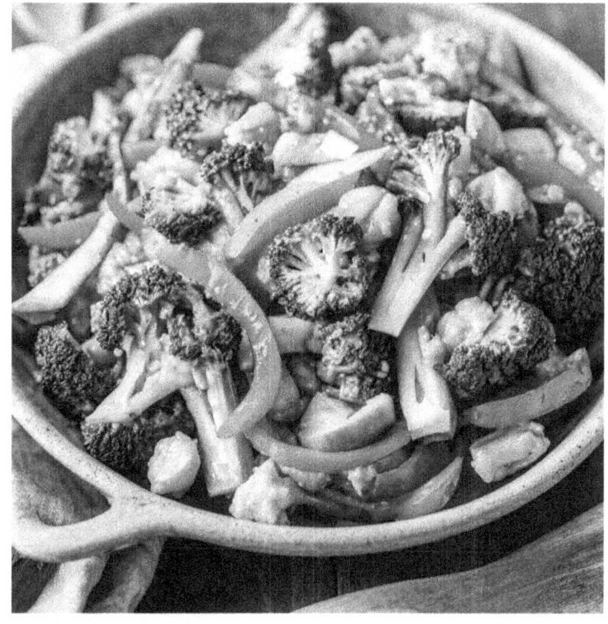

10-WEEK MEAL PLAN

Week 1

Day 1
- Breakfast: Egg and Avocado Salad
- Lunch: Creamed Spinach
- Dinner: Grilled Salmon with Lemon Butter

Day 2
- Breakfast: Spinach and Mushroom Omelette
- Lunch: Cucumber Salad with Sour Cream and Dill
- Dinner: Baked Cod with Herb Crust

Day 3
- Breakfast: Cheese and Herb Frittata
- Lunch: Roasted Cauliflower with Turmeric and Cumin
- Dinner: Tuna Stuffed Avocado

Day 4
- Breakfast: Bacon and Egg Cups
- Lunch: Zucchini Noodles with Pesto
- Dinner: Garlic Butter Shrimp Skewers

Day 5
- Breakfast: Sausage and Pepper Skillet
- Lunch: Eggplant Lasagna
- Dinner: Mussels in Garlic Butter Sauce

Day 6
- Breakfast: Chia Pudding with Coconut Milk
- Lunch: Keto Sushi Rolls
- Dinner: Fish Piccata

Day 7
- Breakfast: Zucchini and Walnut Salad
- Lunch: Creamed Spinach
- Dinner: Salmon Patties with Dill Sauce

Week 2

Day 8
- Breakfast: Greek Yogurt with Nuts and Cinnamon
- Lunch: Cauliflower Rice
- Dinner: Seared Scallops with Bacon

Day 9
- Breakfast: Zucchini and Parmesan Bake
- Lunch: Spaghetti Squash Carbonara
- Dinner: Keto Paella

Day 10
- Breakfast: Bacon and Kale Stir-Fry
- Lunch: Garlic Parmesan Green Beans
- Dinner: Baked Lemon-Garlic Tilapia

Day 11
- Breakfast: Mushroom and Goat Cheese Scramble
- Lunch: Spinach and Feta Stuffed Chicken
- Dinner: Parmesan Crusted Flounder

Day 12
- Breakfast: Broccoli and Cheddar Quiche
- Lunch: Pesto Shrimp with Zoodles
- Dinner: Halibut Steak with Capers

Day 13
- Breakfast: Ricotta and Walnut Cream
- Lunch: Zucchini and Walnut Salad
- Dinner: Keto Fish and Chips

Day 14
- Breakfast: Lemon and Poppy Seed Muffins
- Lunch: Keto Vegetable Stir Fry
- Dinner: Anchovy and Garlic Stuffed Olives

Week 3

Day 15
- Breakfast: Butter-Fried Green Cabbage
- Lunch: Creamed Spinach
- Dinner: Grilled Mackerel with Olive Tapenade

Day 16
- Breakfast: Egg and Olive Tapenade Tartines
- Lunch: Cauliflower Rice
- Dinner: Smoked Trout with Cream Cheese Spread

Day 17
- Breakfast: Cinnamon Bun Smoothie
- Lunch: Eggplant Lasagna
- Dinner: Chicken Thighs with Creamy Garlic Sauce

Day 18
- Breakfast: Cheese and Walnut Balls
- Lunch: Zucchini Noodles with Pesto
- Dinner: Turkey Bacon Wraps

Day 19
- Breakfast: Almond Flour Pancakes
- Lunch: Keto Sushi Rolls
- Dinner: Greek Lemon Chicken Soup

Day 20
- Breakfast: Avocado and Egg Breakfast Pizza
- Lunch: Creamed Spinach
- Dinner: Balsamic Glazed Chicken

Day 21
- Breakfast: Beef and Egg Breakfast Muffins
- Lunch: Zucchini and Walnut Salad
- Dinner: Pesto Chicken Casserole

Week 4

Day 22
- Breakfast: Keto Smoothie
- Lunch: Roasted Cauliflower with Turmeric and Cumin
- Dinner: Smoked Chicken Wings

Day 23
- Breakfast: Ham and Cheese Stuffed Peppers
- Lunch: Eggplant Lasagna
- Dinner: Chicken Liver Pâté

Day 24
- Breakfast: Coconut Flour Crepes
- Lunch: Cauliflower Rice
- Dinner: Chicken Parmesan (Keto Version)

Day 25
- Breakfast: Pumpkin Seed Granola
- Lunch: Spaghetti Squash Carbonara
- Dinner: Shawarma-style Chicken

Day 26
- Breakfast: Cottage Cheese and Flaxseed
- Lunch: Garlic Parmesan Green Beans
- Dinner: Fried Chicken (Almond Flour)

Day 27
- Breakfast: Eggplant and Feta Bake
- Lunch: Zucchini Noodles with Pesto
- Dinner: Baked Haddock with Creamy Dill Sauce

Day 28
- Breakfast: Keto Bagels
- Lunch: Creamed Spinach
- Dinner: Chicken Tikka Masala

Week 5

Day 29
- Breakfast: Cauliflower and Cheese Breakfast Porridge
- Lunch: Roasted Cauliflower with Turmeric and Cumin
- Dinner: Chicken and Mushroom Florentine

Day 30
- Breakfast: Bacon and Kale Stir-Fry
- Lunch: Keto Sushi Rolls
- Dinner: Chicken Skewers with Tzatziki Sauce

Day 31
- Breakfast: Mushroom and Goat Cheese Scramble
- Lunch: Zucchini and Walnut Salad
- Dinner: Turkey Meatballs in Marinara Sauce

Day 32
- Breakfast: Broccoli and Cheddar Quiche
- Lunch: Garlic Parmesan Green Beans
- Dinner: Mustard Roasted Chicken Thighs

Day 33
- Breakfast: Ricotta and Walnut Cream
- Lunch: Creamed Spinach
- Dinner: Garlic Butter Turkey Meatballs

Day 34
- Breakfast: Lemon and Poppy Seed Muffins
- Lunch: Cauliflower Rice
- Dinner: Pesto Shrimp with Zoodles

Day 35
- Breakfast: Butter-Fried Green Cabbage
- Lunch: Zucchini Noodles with Pesto
- Dinner: Fish Piccata

Week 6

Day 36
- Breakfast: Egg and Olive Tapenade Tartines
- Lunch: Spaghetti Squash Carbonara
- Dinner: Creamy Salmon Florentine

Day 37
- Breakfast: Cheese and Walnut Balls
- Lunch: Garlic Parmesan Green Beans
- Dinner: Parmesan Crusted Flounder

Day 38
- Breakfast: Almond Flour Pancakes
- Lunch: Cucumber Salad with Sour Cream and Dill
- Dinner: Halibut Steak with Capers

Day 39
- Breakfast: Avocado and Egg Breakfast Pizza
- Lunch: Zucchini and Walnut Salad
- Dinner: Mussels in Garlic Butter Sauce

Day 40
- Breakfast: Beef and Egg Breakfast Muffins
- Lunch: Keto Vegetable Stir Fry
- Dinner: Keto Paella

Day 41
- Breakfast: Keto Smoothie
- Lunch: Roasted Cauliflower with Turmeric and Cumin
- Dinner: Grilled Mackerel with Olive Tapenade

Day 42
- Breakfast: Ham and Cheese Stuffed Peppers
- Lunch: Cauliflower Rice
- Dinner: Tuna Stuffed Avocado

Week 7

Day 43
- Breakfast: Coconut Flour Crepes
- Lunch: Creamed Spinach
- Dinner: Grilled Salmon with Lemon Butter

Day 44
- Breakfast: Pumpkin Seed Granola
- Lunch: Cucumber Salad with Sour Cream and Dill
- Dinner: Baked Lemon-Garlic Tilapia

Day 45

- Breakfast: Cottage Cheese and Flaxseed
- Lunch: Zucchini Noodles with Pesto
- Dinner: Smoked Trout with Cream Cheese Spread

Day 46

- Breakfast: Eggplant and Feta Bake
- Lunch: Roasted Cauliflower with Turmeric and Cumin
- Dinner: Chicken Thighs with Creamy Garlic Sauce

Day 47

- Breakfast: Keto Bagels
- Lunch: Keto Sushi Rolls
- Dinner: Shawarma-style Chicken

Day 48

- Breakfast: Cauliflower and Cheese Breakfast Porridge
- Lunch: Garlic Parmesan Green Beans
- Dinner: Baked Cod with Herb Crust

Day 49

- Breakfast: Bacon and Kale Stir-Fry
- Lunch: Zucchini and Walnut Salad
- Dinner: Chicken and Mushroom Florentine

Week 8

Day 50

- Breakfast: Mushroom and Goat Cheese Scramble
- Lunch: Creamed Spinach
- Dinner: Pesto Chicken Casserole

Day 51

- Breakfast: Broccoli and Cheddar Quiche
- Lunch: Spaghetti Squash Carbonara
- Dinner: Chicken Liver Pâté

Day 52

- Breakfast: Ricotta and Walnut Cream
- Lunch: Cucumber Salad with Sour Cream and Dill
- Dinner: Smoked Chicken Wings

Day 53

- Breakfast: Lemon and Poppy Seed Muffins
- Lunch: Zucchini Noodles with Pesto
- Dinner: Chicken Tikka Masala

Day 54

- Breakfast: Butter-Fried Green Cabbage
- Lunch: Garlic Parmesan Green Beans
- Dinner: Parmesan Crusted Flounder

Day 55
- Breakfast: Egg and Olive Tapenade Tartines
- Lunch: Zucchini and Walnut Salad
- Dinner: Chicken Skewers with Tzatziki Sauce

Day 56
- Breakfast: Cinnamon Bun Smoothie
- Lunch: Roasted Cauliflower with Turmeric and Cumin
- Dinner: Balsamic Glazed Chicken

Week 9

Day 57
- Breakfast: Cheese and Walnut Balls
- Lunch: Spaghetti Squash Carbonara
- Dinner: Grilled Mackerel with Olive Tapenade

Day 58
- Breakfast: Almond Flour Pancakes
- Lunch: Creamed Spinach
- Dinner: Seared Scallops with Bacon

Day 59
- Breakfast: Avocado and Egg Breakfast Pizza
- Lunch: Keto Vegetable Stir Fry
- Dinner: Mussels in Garlic Butter Sauce

Day 60
- Breakfast: Beef and Egg Breakfast Muffins
- Lunch: Cauliflower Rice
- Dinner: Chicken Parmesan (Keto Version)

Day 61
- Breakfast: Keto Smoothie
- Lunch: Garlic Parmesan Green Beans
- Dinner: Fish Piccata

Day 62
- Breakfast: Ham and Cheese Stuffed Peppers
- Lunch: Cucumber Salad with Sour Cream and Dill
- Dinner: Salmon Patties with Dill Sauce

Day 63
- Breakfast: Coconut Flour Crepes
- Lunch: Zucchini Noodles with Pesto
- Dinner: Keto Paella

Week 10

Day 64

- Breakfast: Pumpkin Seed Granola
- Lunch: Roasted Cauliflower with Turmeric and Cumin
- Dinner: Halibut Steak with Capers

Day 65

- Breakfast: Cottage Cheese and Flaxseed
- Lunch: Garlic Parmesan Green Beans
- Dinner: Baked Haddock with Creamy Dill Sauce

Day 66

- Breakfast: Eggplant and Feta Bake
- Lunch: Zucchini and Walnut Salad
- Dinner: Chicken Liver Pâté

Day 67

- Breakfast: Keto Bagels
- Lunch: Spaghetti Squash Carbonara
- Dinner: Baked Cod with Herb Crust

Day 68

- Breakfast: Cauliflower and Cheese Breakfast Porridge
- Lunch: Cucumber Salad with Sour Cream and Dill
- Dinner: Smoked Trout with Cream Cheese Spread

Day 69

- Breakfast: Bacon and Kale Stir-Fry
- Lunch: Roasted Cauliflower with Turmeric and Cumin
- Dinner: Garlic Butter Shrimp Skewers

Day 70

- Breakfast: Mushroom and Goat Cheese Scramble
- Lunch: Zucchini Noodles with Pesto
- Dinner: Shawarma-style Chicken

Weekly Meal planner+ Journal

	BREAKFAST	LUNCH	DINNER	SNACKS
MON				
TUE				
WED				
THU				
FRI				
SAT				
SUN				

What specific health goals do you hope to achieve by following the Atkins Diet for Epilepsy? (e.g., reduction in seizure frequency, weight management, increased energy levels)

....

....

....

....

....

....

Weekly Meal planner+ Journal

	BREAKFAST	LUNCH	DINNER	SNACKS
MON				
TUE				
WED				
THU				
FRI				
SAT				
SUN				

Describe your current eating habits. What types of foods do you typically eat for breakfast, lunch, and dinner?

....

....

....

....

....

....

Weekly Meal planner + Journal

	BREAKFAST	LUNCH	DINNER	SNACKS
MON				
TUE				
WED				
THU				
FRI				
SAT				
SUN				

How familiar are you with identifying high-carbohydrate foods? List some examples of foods that are high in carbohydrates that you currently eat.

....

....

....

....

....

....

Weekly Meal planner+ Journal

	BREAKFAST	LUNCH	DINNER	SNACKS
MON				
TUE				
WED				
THU				
FRI				
SAT				
SUN				

What challenges do you anticipate facing when transitioning to a low-carbohydrate diet? How do you plan to address these challenges?

....

....

....

....

....

....

Weekly Meal planner+ Journal

	BREAKFAST	LUNCH	DINNER	SNACKS
MON				
TUE				
WED				
THU				
FRI				
SAT				
SUN				

Who in your life can support you in following this diet? How will they help you stay on track?

Weekly Meal planner + Journal

	BREAKFAST	LUNCH	DINNER	SNACKS
MON				
TUE				
WED				
THU				
FRI				
SAT				
SUN				

What are some signs that your body has entered ketosis? How will you monitor these signs?

Weekly Meal planner+ Journal

	BREAKFAST	LUNCH	DINNER	SNACKS
MON				
TUE				
WED				
THU				
FRI				
SAT				
SUN				

What strategies will you use to cope with cravings for high-carbohydrate foods?

Weekly Meal planner+ Journal

	BREAKFAST	LUNCH	DINNER	SNACKS
MON				
TUE				
WED				
THU				
FRI				
SAT				
SUN				

How will you ensure that you are getting enough essential nutrients (vitamins, minerals, fiber) while following the Atkins Diet for Epilepsy?

....

....

....

....

....

Weekly Meal planner+ Journal

	BREAKFAST	LUNCH	DINNER	SNACKS
MON				
TUE				
WED				
THU				
FRI				
SAT				
SUN				

How will you incorporate physical activity into your routine while on the Atkins Diet? Describe the types of exercises you enjoy and how often you plan to do them.

....

....

....

....

....

....

Weekly Meal planner+ Journal

	BREAKFAST	LUNCH	DINNER	SNACKS
MON				
TUE				
WED				
THU				
FRI				
SAT				
SUN				

How will you handle social situations (e.g., dining out, parties) where high-carbohydrate foods might be present? What are some low-carb options you can choose?

....

....

....

....

....

....

Weekly Meal planner+ Journal

	BREAKFAST	LUNCH	DINNER	SNACKS
MON				
TUE				
WED				
THU				
FRI				
SAT				
SUN				

What are your known seizure triggers? How can the Atkins Diet help you manage or avoid these triggers?

After one month on the Atkins Diet for Epilepsy, reflect on your experience. What positive changes have you noticed? What adjustments do you think you need to make to improve your adherence to the diet?

Scan the QR code below to get a surprise bonus